汉英对照

中医养生经典译丛
Chinese-English Translation of Traditional
Chinese Medicine Classics on Health Preservation

三元参赞延寿书

The Book on Prolonging Life by Cultivating Three-Yuan

[元] 李鹏飞 撰
范延妮 韩辉 主译

山东科学技术出版社
·济南·

图书在版编目（CIP）数据

三元参赞延寿书：汉英对照 / （元）李鹏飞撰；范延妮，韩辉主译 . -- 济南：山东科学技术出版社，2024.2

（中医养生经典译丛）

ISBN 978-7-5723-1496-4

Ⅰ . ①三… Ⅱ . ①李… ②范… ③韩… Ⅲ . ①养生（中医）– 中国 – 元代 – 汉、英 Ⅳ . ① R212

中国国家版本馆 CIP 数据核字 (2023) 第 026556 号

三元参赞延寿书

SANYUAN CANZAN YANSHOU SHU

责任编辑：马　祥　夏元枢
装帧设计：孙小杰

主管单位：山东出版传媒股份有限公司
出　版　者：山东科学技术出版社
　　　　　　地址：济南市市中区舜耕路 517 号
　　　　　　邮编：250003　电话：（0531）82098088
　　　　　　网址：www.lkj.com.cn
　　　　　　电子邮件：sdkj@sdcbcm.com
发　行　者：山东科学技术出版社
　　　　　　地址：济南市市中区舜耕路 517 号
　　　　　　邮编：250003　电话：（0531）82098067
印　刷　者：志强云印（山东）智能科技有限公司
　　　　　　地址：济南市历下区八涧堡西路 81 号
　　　　　　邮编：250000　电话：（0531）68657789

规格：16 开（170 mm × 240 mm）
印张：19.25　　字数：230 千
版次：2024 年 2 月第 1 版　印次：2024 年 2 月第 1 次印刷
定价：78.00 元

译 者

主 译 范延妮 韩 辉

副主译 张 洁 张 爽

译 者 王涵琪

丛书序

中医学注重未病先防，倡导不治已病治未病，强调养生的重要性。自《黄帝内经》问世以来，华佗、张仲景、王冰、叶天士等历代医家无不关注养生，或辑先人经验，或创心法要诀，或撰养生精要，护佑中华民族繁衍生息。2021年5月，习近平主席在全球健康峰会上发表题为《携手共建人类卫生健康共同体》的重要讲话，首次提出打造人类卫生健康共同体。中医学作为中华文明的瑰宝，其中凝聚着中华古人智慧的中医养生典籍也应当为全人类健康福祉服务。为此，我们精选《养老奉亲书》《三元参赞延寿书》《养性延命录》《饮膳正要》等经典养生古籍并译为英文，是为"中医养生经典译丛"，以飨读者。

《养老奉亲书》，宋代陈直撰，包括饮食调治、形证脉候、医药扶持、性气好嗜、宴处起居、食治老人诸疾方等内容，主要论述老年保健、四时摄养措施、疾病预防理论及治疗方法，主张老人有病，先食疗之，未愈则命药疗之，饮食宜温热熟饮、忌黏硬生冷，药饵宜用扶持之法，对老年养生具有指导意义。

《三元参赞延寿书》，元代李鹏飞撰，将人之寿命分为天元、地元、人元。"天元之寿"为"精神不耗者得之"，讨论人欲生殖，提出欲不可绝、欲不可早、欲不可纵、欲不可强、欲有所忌、欲有所避等主张；"地元之寿"为"起居有常者得之"，讨论情绪与起居，包括调情绪、慎起居、顺天时等；"人元之寿"为"饮食有度者得之"，讨论健康饮食，提出许多饮食养生方法。

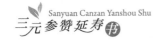

《养性延命录》，南北朝陶弘景撰，辑录上自炎黄、下至魏晋的养生理论与方法，分上、下两卷，包括《教诫篇》《食诫篇》《杂诫忌禳害祈善篇》《服气疗病篇》《导引按摩篇》《御女损益篇》六篇，分别讲述养生理论、饮食宜忌、日常起居、行气之术、导引按摩和房中术，是道教史上对养生术的一次大总结，反映了道教学者对益寿延年的重视。

《饮膳正要》，元代忽思慧撰，是一部营养学专著，共三卷：卷一是诸般禁忌、聚珍异馔；卷二是诸般汤煎、食疗诸病及食物相反中毒等；卷三是米谷品、兽品、禽品、鱼品、果菜品和料物等。内容主要阐述各种饮馔的性味与滋补作用，还包括医疗卫生，历代名医的验方、秘方和具有蒙古族饮食特点的各种肉、乳食品，为我国现存最早的饮食卫生和食疗专书，对研究中医药，尤其是蒙古医药科技史具有重要的意义。

译者团队选取四部典籍的权威版本为蓝本，并参照多个通行本进行校勘，依据世界卫生组织、世界中医药学会联合会等颁布的标准翻译基本名词术语，力争最大限度理解和再现典籍原文内容，为中医海外从业者和研究者开展中医理论溯源和传承创新提供研究基础。

由于译者水平有限，加之时间紧张，错讹之处敬请读者批评指正。

译　者

2023 年 3 月

翻译说明

1. 本次所译的《三元参赞延寿书》，以中医古籍出版社影印清人精抄《寿养丛书》为汉语底本，并参考了多个通行本。

2. 典籍书名，采用音译的方法翻译，括号中附以中文和英语翻译，音译以词为单位。例如《史记》译为 *Shi Ji*（《史记》，*Historical Records*）。

3. 中草药名称的翻译采取"四保险"的翻译方法，即每个本草名称均按拼音、汉字、英语和拉丁语的方式进行翻译，例如熟地黄译为 Shudihuang［熟地黄，Prepared Rehmannia Root, Radix Rehmanniae Preparata］。

4. 书中涉及的药物剂量单位属元代的度量衡单位，与现代度量衡单位有别。均采用音译方法，其基本形式和释义如下：

传统剂量单位	公制剂量单位	音译形式
分	9.5 克	Fen
钱	3.8 克	Qian
两	38 克	Liang
斤	608 克	Jin
合	100.3 毫升	He
升	100 3 毫升	Sheng
斗	100 30 毫升	Dou
寸	3.5 厘米	Cun
尺	35 厘米	Chi

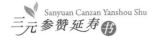

Translation Specification

1. The translation of *San Yuan Can Zan Yan Shou Shu* （《三元参赞延寿书》, *A Book on Prolonging Life by Cultivating Three-Yuan*）takes its Chinese photocopy from *Shou Yang Cong Shu* （《寿养丛书》, *The Series of Books on Longevity and Health Preservation*）published by Traditional Chinese Medicine Ancient Books Publishing House as the master copy, and also refers to many current versions.

2. The names of ancient books are transliterated from Chinese characters into Pinyin in phrases, with the Chinese name and English version in bracket. For instance,《史记》is translated as *Shi Ji* （《史记》, *Historical Records*）.

3. For the translation of herbal names, the "Four Assurance Method" is adopted, namely, every herbal name is translated in the way that its four forms are listed in the sequence of Pinyin, Chinese character, English and Latin. For instance, "熟地黄" is translated as Shudihuang［熟地黄, Prepared Rehmannia Root, Radix Rehmanniae Preparata］.

4. The dosage units involved in this book is in accordance with those in the Yuan Dynasty, quite different with modern ones, so they are transliterated into Pinyin. Refer to the table below:

Traditional dosage unit	Metric dosage unit	Pinyin
分	9.5 克	Fen
钱	3.8 克	Qian
两	38 克	Liang
斤	608 克	Jin
合	100.3 毫升	He
升	100 3 毫升	Sheng
斗	100 30 毫升	Dou
寸	3.5 厘米	Cun
尺	35 厘米	Chi

本书为山东中医药大学英语专业建设成果；山东中医药大学"中医话语特征与中医翻译"青年科研创新团队成果；山东中医药大学中医养生学学科建设与专业建设成果。

序

Preface

  黄帝问岐伯曰："余闻上古之人，春秋皆度百岁而动作不衰，今时之人，年至半百而动作皆衰，时世异耶？人将失之耶？"岐伯对曰："上古之人，其知道者，法于阴阳，和于术数，食饮有节，起居有常，不妄作劳，故能形与神俱，而尽终其天年。今时之人不然也。以酒为浆，以妄为常，以欲竭其精。以耗散其真，不知持满，不时御神，务快其心，逆于生乐，故半百而衰也。"又曰："知之则强，不知则老，知则耳目聪明，身体轻健，老者复壮，寿命与天地无穷。"此仆养生延寿之书所由作欤。

  Huangdi asked Qibo, "I am told that people in ancient times all could live for one hundred years without any signs of senility. But people nowadays begin to become old at the age of fifty. Is it due to the changes of environment or the violation of the way to preserve health?" Qibo answered, "The sages in ancient times who knew the principle for cultivating health followed the rules of Yin and Yang, and adjusted the ways to cultivate health. They were moderate in diet, regular in lifestyle, and far away from

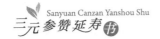

overstrain. That is why they could maintain a desirable harmony between the spirit and the body, enjoying good health and a long life. People nowadays, on the contrary, just behave oppositely. They drink wine as thin rice gruel, regard wrong as right, and seek sexual pleasure after drinking. As a result, their essential qi is exhausted and genuine qi is consumed. They seldom take measures to keep a balance of essential qi and to regulate the spirit properly, often giving themselves to sensual pleasure. Being irregular in daily life, they begin to become old even at the age of fifty." Then he added, "Those who understand how to cultivate health enjoy good health while those who do not know how to preserve health cannot escape from premature aging. Those who understand how to cultivate health have sufficient vitality with normal hearing and eyesight, lively and strong body, and they can still enjoy a healthy body even at an elderly age. So they can prolong their life and enjoy a happy and natural life span." This is the reason why I wrote this book about health cultivation and longevity prolonging.

所谓养生者，既非炉鼎之诀，使惮于金石之费者不能为；又非吐纳之术，使牵于事物之变者不暇为。郭橐驼有云："驼非能使人寿且孳也，以能顺人之天，而致其性焉耳。"仆此书，不过顺乎人之天，皆日用而不可缺者。故他书可有也，可无也。此书则可有，也必不可无也。

Health cultivation, as it is called, is neither to make immortal pills in stove and tripod which may hold people back by the high cost of metal and stone, nor to practice exhalation and inhalation which is conditional and time consuming for busy people. Guo Tuotuo once said, "I myself can not prolong life and promote reproduction for people. My method is to follow the law of nature and correspond to it." Similarly, this book tries to understand and follow the nature of human beings and explores health cultivation methods indispensable to daily life. Therefore, different with other books that can be necessary or unnecessary, this book is a must for people to preserve their health.

　　仆生甫二周，而生母迁于淮北，壮失所在，哀号奔走淮东西者，凡三年。天悯其衷，见母于蕲之罗田。自是岁于涉淮。一日道出庞居士旧址，遇一道人，绿发童颜，问姓，曰："宫也。"问所之，曰："采药。"与语移日，清越可喜，同宿焉。道人夜坐达旦，问其齿，九十余矣。诘其所以寿？曰："子闻三元之说乎？"时匆匆不暇叩。后十年戊辰，试太学至礼部，少憩飞来峰下，忽复遇其人，貌不减旧。始异之，携手同饮。因诘向语。道人曰："此常理耳。"余稽手请之。曰："人之寿，天元六十，地元六十，人元六十，共一百八十岁。不知戒慎，则日加损焉。精神不固，则天元之寿减矣；谋为过当，则地元之寿减矣；饮食不节，则人元之寿减矣。当宝啬而不知所爱，当禁忌而不知所避，神日以耗，病日以来，而寿日以促矣。其说皆具见于黄帝岐伯《素问》、老聃、庄周及名医书中，其与孔孟无异。子归以吾说求之，无他术也。"复为余细析其说，且遗以二图，余再拜谢。蚤夜以思之，前之所为，其可悔者多矣。于是以其说，搜诸书，集而成编，以自警焉。

When I was two weeks old, my mother moved to the Northern Huaihe Area and I lost contact with her for the whole childhood. I spent three years in search of her around the eastern and western parts of Huai area, and

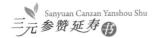

blessed by God, found her finally in Luotian of Qi prefecture. Since then, I went there to visit my mother once a year. One day, I met a Taoist with green hair and ruddy complexion in the former site of lay Buddhist Pang. I asked his surname and he said Gong. I asked where he was going and he said to collect herbs. We had a pleasant talk and spent the night together. He sat up the whole night and said he was over nineties when asked about his age. I asked the secret for his longevity and he said, " Have you heard the theory of Three Yuan?" I did not inquire about the details that time in haste. Ten years later, I met the Daoist again on the way to be interviewed from the Imperial College to the Ministry of Rites when I took a rest at the foot of the Feilai mountain. He was the same as before and I was very surprised, so I invited him to drink together and asked the secret. He said, "This is the universal law." I knelt down and asked for more information. He said, "People are supposed to live 180 years old, which consists of 60 years granted by heaven, 60 years by earth and 60 years by human being. The longevity may be shortened if people do not abstain from taboos. The longevity granted by heaven may be shortened if the essential qi is not consolidated; the longevity granted by earth may be shortened if people are over thinking; the longevity granted by human being may be shortened if the diet is improper. The spirit may be exhausted, the disease may occur and the longevity may be shortened gradually if people are confused when facing treasures and unable to elude when facing taboos. These remarks can also be found in *Su Wen*（《素问》, *Plain Questions*）and the books written by Lao Zi, Zhuang Zi and other famous physicians, which are quite similar with the ideas of Confucius and

Mencius. You can explore the methods for longevity based on my remarks when you go back home and there is no other way to realize it. " Then he explained in detail and left two illustrations to me and I bowed to him to show my gratitude. Then I reflected day and night on the regrettable practices of my previous life and started to search for relevant books and compile them for self warning.

仆年七十，父年且九十一矣，蒙恩免役侍奉，他无以仰报，明时愿锓诸梓，与众共之，庶读者详焉。不敢以父母遗体行殆，安乐寿考，以泳太平，似于天朝好生之德，不为无补云旨。

This year I am 70 years old and my father is 91 years old. Thanks to the kindness of the emperor, I am exempt from the duty and able to attend upon my father at home. There is nothing I can do in return but to print and publish the book and let the readers benefit from it. I dare not risk the body given by parents in danger but I can contribute to the happiness and longevity of the people by this book, with the purpose of conforming to the emperor's virtue of cherishing life and benefiting the society.

至元辛卯岁菊月吉旦九华澄心老人

李鹏飞

Li Pengfei

The first day of the ninth lunar month, 1291

目　录

Contents

卷之首

人　说

On Human Being ·························· 001

卷之一

天元之寿

Prolonging Life by Cultivating Tian Yuan ·················· 008

欲不可绝

The Moderation of Sexual Activity ·················· 012

欲不可早

The Right Age for Sexual Activity ·················· 016

欲不可纵

The Proper Restraint on Sexual Activity ·················· 018

欲不可强

Sexual Activity Kept within One's Capability ·················· 025

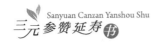
欲有所忌

Taboos about Sexual Activity ································· 027

欲有所避

Conditions to Keep off for Sexual Activity ··········· 032

嗣续有方

Proper Methods to Conceive ····························· 036

妊娠所忌

Taboos during Pregnancy ································· 039

婴儿所忌

Taboos for Baby ··· 042

卷之二

地元之寿

Prolonging Life by Cultivating Di Yuan ················· 044

养生之道

Ways to Preserve Health ································· 046

喜乐

Joy ··· 049

忿怒

Anger ··· 052

悲哀

Sorrow ·· 055

思虑

Thought ··· 057

忧愁

Anxiety ·· 061

愁泣

Weeping ··· 063

惊恐

Fright and Fear ·· 065

憎爱

Hatred and Preference ································ 068

视听

Vision and Hearing ··································· 070

疑惑

Suspicion ··· 074

谈笑

Talking and Laughing ································ 077

津睡

Saliva ·· 079

起居

Daily Life ··· 082

行立

Walking and Standing ································ 088

坐卧

Sitting and Lying ····································· 092

沐浴洗面

Bathing and Washing Face ·························· 097

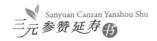

栉发

Hair Combing ················· 101

大小腑

Urination and Defecation ··········· 105

衣著汗

Clothing ········· 108

天时避忌

Taboos Related with Climate ············ 112

四时调摄

Health Preservation in the Four Seasons ·········· 115

旦暮避忌

Taboos Concerning Dawn and Dusk ··········· 122

杂忌

Miscellaneous Taboos ············· 125

卷之三

人元之寿

Prolonging Life by Cultivating Ren Yuan ············ 128

五味

The Five Flavors ············· 130

饮食

Diet ·········· 136

食物

Food ·········· 155

果实

Fruits ·· 156

米谷

Grains ·· 168

菜蔬

Vegetables ·· 177

飞禽

Fowls ··· 196

走兽

Beasts ·· 207

鱼类

Fishes ·· 229

虫类

Insects ·· 251

卷之四

神仙救世却老还童真诀

The Pithy Formula of the Immortals Saving the World and

　　Renewing Youth ······································· 257

滋补有药

Medicines for Nourishment ···················· 262

导引有法

Guiding Exercise Methods for Health Preservation ·············· 265

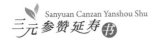

神仙警世

Cautionary Remarks from Immortals ···················· 272

阴德延寿论

On Life Extension by Hidden Virtue ···················· 275

函三为一歌并图

The Song and Diagram of Three-Yuan-in-One ················ 281

还元图

The Diagram of Restoring Vitality ························ 283

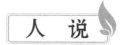

人　说

On Human Being

　　天地之间人为贵，然囿于形而莫知其所以贵也。头圆象天，足方象地，目象日月，毛发肉骨象山林土石，呼为风，呵为露，喜而景星庆云，怒而震霆迅雷，血液流润，而江河淮海。至于四肢之四时，五脏之五行，六腑之六律，若是者，吾身天地同流也。岂不贵乎？

　　Human beings are regarded as the most valuable creatures in nature, but their value is not fully recognized due to the confinement of their physical structures. For human beings, their round heads may be analogized to the heaven, their square feet to the earth, their eyes to the sun and the moon, their hairs, muscles and bones to the mountains, forests, soils and rocks, their exhalation to the wind, their breath to the dew, their joy to auspicious signs like colored cloud and propitious star, their anger to the thunder and lightening, their blood to the river, stream and sea. Just as it is supposed to be, the limbs correspond to the four seasons, the five zang-organs correspond to the five elements, the six fu-organs correspond to the six pitches of music, so the whole body correspond to the nature. Aren't human beings valuable?

按藏教父母及子相感，业神入胎，地水火风，众缘和合，渐得长生。一七日如藕根；二七日如稠酪；三七日如鞋袜；四七日如温石；五七日有风触胎，名摄提，头及两臂胫，五种相现；六七日有风，名旋转，两手足四相现；七七及八七日，手足十指二十四相现；九七日眼、耳、鼻、口及下二穴、大小便处九种相现；十七日有风，名普门吹，令坚实及生五脏；十一七日上下气通；十二七日大小肠生；十三七日渐知饥渴，饮食滋味，皆从脐入；十四七日身前身后，左右二边各生五十条脉；十五七日又生二十条脉，一身之中共有八百吸气之脉，至是皆具；十六七日有风，名甘露，安置两眼，通诸出入息气；十七七日有风，名毛拂，能令眼、耳、鼻、口、咽喉、胸臆一切合入之处，皆得通滑；十八七日有风，名无垢，能令六根清净；十九七日眼、耳、鼻、舌四根成就，得种报曰身命意；二十七日有风，名坚固，二脚、二手、二十指节至，一身二百大骨及诸小骨，一切皆生；二十一日有风，名生起，能令生肉；二十二七日有风，名浮流，能令生血；二十三七日生皮；二十四七日皮肤光悦；二十五七日血肉滋润；二十六七日发毛爪甲皆与脉通；二十七七日发毛爪甲悉皆生就；二十八七日生屋宇园池河等八想；二十九七日各随自业，或鳖或白；三十七日鳖白想现；三十一七日至三十四七日渐得增长；三十五七日肢体具足；三十六七日不乐住腹；三十七七日生不净臭秽，黑暗三想；三十八七日有风，名蓝花，能令长伸两臂，转身向下，次越下风，能令足上首下，以向生门。是时也，万神必唱，恭而生男，万神必唱，奉而生女。至于五脏六腑，筋骨髓脑，皮肤血肢，精脏水脏，二万八千形景，一万二千精光，三万六千出入，八万四千毛窍，莫不各有其神以主之。然则人身，岂易得哉？鞠育之恩，又岂浅浅哉？夫以天地父母之恩，生此不易得之身，至可贵，至可宝者。

Tibetan Buddhism believes that the birth of a baby is a result of the intercourse of its parents. It is noted that Karma God enters the womb, then women become pregnant. The fetus will start to grow when earth, water, fire, air and all the other elements are in a harmonious state. The fetus is shaped like a lotus root by the first week, a thick piece of cheese by the second, a shoe by the third, and a piece of serpentine by the fourth. By the fifth week, touched by the wind named Sheti, the fetus develops its head and four limbs. By the sixth and seventh week, touched by the wind named Xuanzhuan, the fetus develops its hands and feet. By the seventh and eighth week, beyond the hands and feet, the fetus develops its fingers and toes. By the ninth week, eyes, ears, nostrils, mouth, urinary organ and anus are developed. By the tenth week, touched by the wind named Pumenchui, the fetus becomes solid and develops the five internal organs. By the eleventh week, qi flows freely through the fetus. By the twelfth week, the fetus develops its large and small intestine. By the thirteenth week, the fetus gradually develops the sense of hunger and thirst. And the nutrients are transported to the fetus through the umbilical cord. By the fourteenth week, fifty meridians are formed on the front, back, left and right sides of the fetus. By the fifteenth week, twenty more meridians are developed. By then, the fetus has a total of

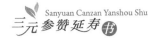

eight hundred meridians through which qi can flow. By the sixteenth week, touched by the wind named Ganlu, the fetus develops its eyes. And all the pores start to ventilate. By the seventeenth week, touched by the wind named Maofu, the body parts of the fetus like eyes, ears, nose, mouth, throat and chest are interconnected and unobstructed. By the eighteenth week, touched by the wind named Wugou, the six roots of the fetus, including eyes, ears, nose, tongue, body and mind are refreshed. By the nineteenth week, the fetus's eyes, nose, ears and tongue are further developed. The retribution is manifested by the body, mind and life. By the twentieth week, touched by the wind named Jiangu, the fetus develops bones of feet, hands and knuckles, as well as the two hundred large bones and many small bones all over the body. By the twenty-first week, touched by the wind named Shengqi, the fetus develops its flesh. By the twenty-second week, touch by the wind named Fuliu, the fetus develops its blood. By the twenty-third week, the fetus develops its skin. By the twenty-fourth week, its skin becomes smooth. By the twenty-fifth week, the blood and flesh become moist. By the twenty-sixth week, the fetus's hairs and nails are connected with meridians. By the twenty-seventh week, its hairs and nails are formed. By the twenty-eighth week, the fetus develops ideas about eight things, including houses, gardens, pools and rivers. By the twenty-ninth week, the fetus starts to follow its karma, either good or bad. By the thirtieth week, the thoughts of goodness or evil start to appear. During the thirty-first to thirty-fourth week, the fetus gradually grows. By the thirty-fifth week, the fetus's body and limbs are fully developed. By the thirty-sixth week, the frequency of fetal movement increases. By the thirty-seventh week, the fetus develops impurity, stink dirt and three kinds of dark ideas. By the thirty-eighth week, touched by the wind named Lanhua, the fetus stretches its arms and turns around with its feet up and head down along the direction of the wind. Thus, it's ready to be born. By then, all Gods will extol the birth of a son or a daughter. As for the five zang-organs, the six fu-organs, the bone and sinew, the marrow and brain, the skin and limbs, the kidney, along with about 28,000 shapes of scene, 12,000 looks, 36,000 ways of exiting and entering of qi and 84,000 pores, they are all governed by their own spirit. Therefore, how could the human body be so easily formed? How could the parents' upbringing be valued too much? It's a gift from the nature and parents that one can conquer so much to obtain its body. In this way, human beings are indeed the most valuable creatures ever.

　　五福，一曰寿而已。既得其寿，则富贵利达，致君泽民，光前振后，凡所以掀揭宇宙者，皆可为也。盖身者，亲之身。轻其身是轻其亲矣，安可不知所守，以全天与之寿，而有以尽事亲之大乎？或曰：婴孺之流，天真未剖，禁忌饮食又无所犯，有至夭枉者，何欤？曰：此父母之过也。为父母者，或阳盛阴虚；或阴盛阳虚；或七情郁于内；或八邪袭于外；或母因胎寒而饵暖药；或父阴萎而饵丹药；或胎元既充，淫欲未已，如花伤培，结子不实。既产之后，禀赋怯弱，调养又失其宜，骄惜太过。睡思既浓，尚令咀嚼。火合既暖，犹令饮酌。厚衾重覆，且令衣着，抚背拍衣，风从内作。指物为虫，惊因戏谑，危坐放手，我笑渠恶，欲令喜笑，肋胁指齖。雷鸣击鼓，且与掩耳。眠卧过时，不令早起。饮食饱饫，不与戒止。睡卧当风，恐吓神鬼。如此等事，不一而已。斯言也，演山

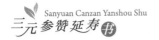
省翁之至言也。父母者因是而鉴之，则后嗣流芳，同此一寿，岂不伟欤。

The first of the five blessings is longevity. As long as a person can live a long life, he will be rich and wealthy, thus he will contribute his own knowledge and talents to serve the society, the country, and even the whole world. He can do anything to explore the world and the universe. The human body is originated from the parents and belongs to the parents. People who neglect their own bodies actually neglect their parents. How could people not know the ways to take care of themselves to live to the age granted by heaven and perform their duty of filial piety to parents? Someone says: There are people like young children, very naive and unable to distinguish things, who are fed with proper diet but still die prematurely. Why? The answer is that it is the parents' fault. For parents, there may exist the following problems: yang exuberance and yin deficiency, yin exuberance and yang deficiency; seven emotions stagnated in the body; invasion of eight excesses from the outside; the mother's taking of warm medicinals to treat fetal cold, the father's taking of pellets because of sexual dysfunction; damage to the formed fetus because of parents' sexual life in pregnancy just like a flower unable to bear fruits due to injury to the root. After the baby is born, he is poor in natural endowment, and nursed improperly and over indulgently. He is allowed to chew when still sleepy, to take hot beverage when in warm room, to wear more clothes when covered in thick quilt. He is attacked by internal wind due to patting on the back, frightened by objects that are teasingly pointed as insects. He is unpleasant to be let go when sitting in dangerous places and to be tickled for fun. He is protected by covering his ears when there is thunder and drumming, allowed to get up late when his sleep is enough, permitted to eat more when he is full, invaded by wind and frightened by ghost when in sleep. Such kind of things can not be listed all here. This is true of what Master Yan Shansheng said. Parents need to warn themselves against these behaviors and leave a good reputation to their offspring. Then all of them will have a good life and obtain longevity. Isn't that a great thing?

明·钱塘胡文焕（德父）校

Collated by Hu Wenhuan from Qiantang County of Ming Dynasty

天元之寿 精神不耗者得之

Prolonging Life by Cultivating Tian Yuan

Those Who Don't Exhaust the Essence and Spirit Can Achieve It

男女居室，人之大伦，独阳不生，独阴不成，人道有不可废者。

It is an essential ethic for man and woman to live together and have sexual activity. Man pertains to yang and woman to yin. Yang can not exist without yin and vice versa. This is something that can not be neglected for the development of human beings.

庄周乃曰："人之可畏者，衽席之间，不知戒者过也。"

Zhuang Zhou（a representative of Taoist philosophy in the Warring States Period）said, "The most terrifying thing for people is to engage themselves in sexual indulgence without restraint."

盖此身与造化同流，左为肾，属水；右为命门，属火。

The reason is that the body corresponds with the law of nature. On its left is the kidney, which pertains to water in the five elements; on its right is the life-gate, which pertains to fire in the five elements.

阳生于子，火实藏之，犹北方之有龟蛇也。

Yang originates from male and is hidden in the fire, just as the turtle and snake[1] in the north.

膀胱为左肾之腑，三焦为右肾之腑。三焦有脂膜如掌大，正与膀胱相对，有二白脉，自中而出，夹脊而上，贯于脑。上焦在膻中，内应心；中焦在中脘，内应脾；下焦在脐，下即肾间，动气分布，人身方其湛寂。欲念不兴，精气散于三焦，荣华百脉。及欲想一起，欲火炽然，翕撮三焦，精气流溢，并从命门输泻而去。可畏哉！

Inside the body, the bladder is the fu-organ related with the kidney on the left, and the triple energizer is the fu-organ related with the kidney on the right. The triple energizers contain the lipid membrane as big as the palm opposite to the bladder, from which there are two vessels flowing upward through the spine to the brain. The upper energizer is located in the center of chest, which corresponds to the heart; the middle energizer is located in the middle abdomen, which corresponds to the spleen; the lower energizer is located in the umbilicus, which corresponds to the kidney. When qi moves

---

[1] It is said that tortoises and snakes in nature cannot survive alone and are always entangled; water and fire in human body cannot exist alone but interact and depend on each other.

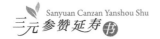
smoothly in the body, the dynamic equilibrium is maintained. When the desire is not aroused, the essential qi disperses in the triple energizers and nourishes the vessels. When the desire is aroused and the heat it produces will cause the opening and contraction of the three energizers and then the flowing out of the essential qi everywhere, which may be consumed and purged out from the gate of life. What a terrible thing it is!

嗟夫，元气有限，人欲无涯，火生于木，祸发必克，尾闾不禁，沧海以竭。少之时，血气未定，既不能守夫子在色之戒。及其老也，则当寡欲闲心。又不能明列子养生之方，吾不知其可也。

Oops! A person's vitality is limited, but his desire is limitless. A person's life is like the fire generated from wood, any disorder will restrain the longevity; A person's life is like the water in sea, repeated appearance of lower reaches will dry up it. When a person is young, he is prosperous in vigour and can not restrain himself from the sexual desires from which the Confucius has warned against; when he is elderly, he should pursue an abstinent and leisurely life. If he has no idea about the methods to cultivate health put forward by various scholars, I do not know how he can live a long life.

麻衣道人曰："天地人等列三才，人得中道，可以学圣贤，可以学神仙。"况人之数，多于天地万物之数。但今之人不修人道，贪爱嗜欲，其数消灭，只与物同也。所以有老、病、夭、伤之患。鉴乎此，必知所以自重而可以得天元之寿矣。

A Daoist in sackcloth said, "The heaven, the earth, and the human being are three life levels in nature. Being in the middle path, human being can learn from sages and men of virtue and immortals. Besides, the population of human being is far more than the total number of other creatures in the world. However, it is a pity that human beings do not follow the living rules in society and the population is diminished to the same as the other creatures due to their greed and desires. Consequently, there exist various sufferings like aging, disease, premature death and wound. So it is essential to know how to preserve health and live a natural longevity.

欲不可绝

The Moderation of Sexual Activity

　　黄帝曰：一阴一阳之谓道，偏阴偏阳之谓疾。曰：两者不和，若春无秋，若冬无夏，因而和之，是谓圣度。圣人不绝和合之道，但贵于闭密，以守天真也。

The Yellow Emperor said, "The way of nature is composed of yin and yang, and the imbalance between them leads to disease." He also said, "The disharmony between yin and yang is just like a flowering spring without a fruitful autumn, a cold winter without a hot summer. Therefore, the harmonious coexistence of yin and yang is a normal and natural law. The ancient sage never goes against the harmonious coexistence of yin and yang, but attaches importance to the moderation of sexual activity to protect the essential qi."

　　《素女》曰：人年二十者，四日一泄；三十者，八日一泄；四十者，十六日一泄；五十者，二十日一泄。

It is narrated in *Su Nv* （《素女经》, *The Maiden Scriptures*）that people at the age of 20s should ejaculate once every four days; those at the age of 30s should ejaculate once every eight days; those at the age of 40s should ejaculate once every 16 days; those at the age of 50s should ejaculate once every 20 days.

此法语也。所禀者厚，食饮多，精力健，或少过其度。譬之井焉，源深流长，虽随汲随满，犹惧其竭也。若所禀者薄，元气本弱，又食减精耗，顾强而为之，是怯夫而试冯妇之术，适以劘虎牙耳。

Of course, this is just a general rule. If a person is born with strong endowments who has good appetite and vigorous energy, he can outdo the limitation mentioned above. But he should be cautious at the same time for fear of the depletion of essence just as a deep well, whose water can be refilled after frequent taking, still needs to ensure its supply at the long term. If a person is born with a weak endowment who has feeble vitality, poor appetite and exhausted essence, he should not behave narrowly with difficulty. Otherwise, he is just like a coward resuming his old trade as Feng Fu of the Jin Dynasty who forgot his decision to be a charitable person and started to fight with tiger again.

《素女》曰：人年六十者，常闭精勿泄，若气力尚壮盛者，亦不可强忍久而不泄，致生痈疾。

Su Nv（《素女经》, *The Maiden Scriptures*）says: When a person is over 60 years old, he should stop sexual activity to protect the essence from losing. However, if he is still strong enough, he should not restrain himself too much to avoid disorder and carbuncle.

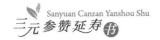

彭祖曰：男不可无女，女不可无男。若念头正直，无可思者，大住长年也。又曰：人能一月再泄精，一岁二十四泄，得寿二百岁。

Peng Zu (an ancient Daoist famous for his longevity) said, "A man cannot live without a woman, and a woman cannot live without a man. If they possess moderate and appropriate desire, they can enjoy a long life." Peng Zu also said, "If a person has sexual activity twice a month and 24 times a year, he can achieve a life span of 200 years."

《名医论》曰：思欲无穷，所愿不得，意淫于外，为白淫而下，因是入房太甚，宗筋纵弛。

Ming Yi Lun (《名医论》, *Famous Physicians' Discussion*) says: If one's desire for sexual activity is not satisfied, it would be discharged out in the form of seminal emission. This is because of the lassitude of male external genitals due to the overindulgence in sexual activity.

书云：男子以精为主，女子以血为主，故精盛则思室，血盛则怀胎。若孤阳绝阴，独阴无阳，欲心炽而不遂，则阴阳交争，乍寒乍热，久而为劳。

The present book says: Essence is critical for men and blood for women. When the essence is sufficient, men will think about sexual activity; when the blood is sufficient, women will conceive babies. Yang and yin, just as men and women, can not live without each other. If they can not have normal sexual activity, there will be imbalance between yin and yang and alternate cold and heat, resulting in overexertion finally.

富家子唐靖，疮发于阴至烂，道人周守真曰："病得之欲泄而不可泄也。"《史记》

济北王侍人韩女，病腰背痛，寒热。仓公曰："病得之欲男子不可得也。"

Tang Jing, a son of a wealthy family, developed sore carbuncle on his genitals, which had festered. A Taoist named Zhou Shouzhen said, "The cause of this disease is the desire to have sexual activity is not satisfied. " It is recorded in *Shi Ji*（《史记》, *Historical Records*）that the maid of the King of Jibei, surnamed Han, suffered from lumbago and backache, cold and heat. Cang Gong, a famous physician of the Western Han Dynasty, said, "The cause of this disease is the desire to have sexual activity is not satisfied. "

欲不可早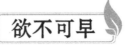

The Right Age for Sexual Activity

齐大夫褚澄曰：羸女则养血，宜及时而嫁；弱男则节色，宜待壮而婚。

Chu Cheng, a physician in the Southern Dynasty, said, "The emaciated young woman should get married timely when her blood is nourished well; the weak young man should get married timely when he is strong and vigorous enough after proper continence."

书云：男子破阳太早，则伤其精气；气女破阴太早，则伤其血脉。

The present book says: A man who starts sexual intercourse too early will get the essential qi damaged; a woman who starts sexual intercourse too early will get the blood and vessels damaged.

书云：精未通而御女，以通其精，则五体有不满之处，异日有不状之疾。

The present book says: If a young man has sexual activity before the due time, there will be some underdevelopment in various parts of the body and indescribable diseases in the future.

书云：未笄之女，天癸始至，已近男色，阴气早泄，未完而伤。

The present book says: If a young woman who just starts to have menstruation bu does not reach the hairpin stage（marriageable age）has sexual activity, the yin qi will be discharged and damaged.

书云：童男室女积想在心，思虑过当，多致苛损，男则神色先散，女则月水先闭。

The present book says: If virgin boys and girls think too much of sexual activity, they will suffer from impairment severely. The boys may look dispirited and sluggish and the girls may suffer from amenorrhoea.

欲不可纵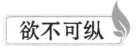

The Proper Restraint on Sexual Activity

《黄庭经》曰：长生至慎房中急，何为使作令神泣。

Huang Ting Jing（《黄庭经》, *The Classic of the Yellow Yard*）says: To prolong life, the first thing to be cautious about is to have restraint on sexual activity to avoid the eagerness and overindulgence. Why do people look for trouble like this?

彭祖曰：上士异床，中士异被。服药千裹，不如独卧。

Peng Zu said, "To avoid sexual overindulgence, the wise sleeps in separate beds and the average sleeps with different quilts. Sleeping alone is better than taking hundreds of formulas of medicinals."

老君曰：情欲出于五内，魂定魄静，生也；情欲出于胸臆，精散神惑，死也。

Laojun said, "If the sexual desire comes from the internal organs and physical needs, it is beneficial for health because it can pacify the spirit and calm the mind. If the sexual desire comes from the subjective will, it may cause death because it can consume the essence and confuse the mind."

彭祖曰：“美色妖丽，娇妾盈房，以致虚损之祸，知此可以长生。”

Peng Zu said, "Having too many beautiful and charming wives and concubines tend to cause sexual overindulgence and may lead to deficiency and damage to the body. Knowing this fact can help to prolong life."

《阴符经》曰：淫声美色，破骨之斧锯也。世之人若不能秉灵烛以照迷情，持慧剑以割爱欲，则流浪生死之海，害生于恩也。

Yinfu Jing（《黄帝阴符经》, *Huangdi's Canon of Implicit Conjunction*）says: Obscene music and attractive women are destructive just like axe and saw for cutting bones. If people can't hold a soul candle to perceive the puzzling emotions and hold the sword of wisdom to cut off their sexual desire, they will wander in the sea of unpredictable misery and be damaged by the harmful preference.

全元起曰：乐色不节则精耗，轻用不止则精散，圣人爱精，重施髓满骨坚。

Quan Yuanqi says, "The essence may be consumed if people have no restraint on their sexual desire; the essence may be exhausted if people have no end in sexual activity. Those with superb intelligence know how to cherish the essence and strengthen the marrow and bones."

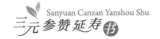
书云：年高之时，血气既弱，觉阳事辄盛，必慎而抑之。不可纵心竭意，一度不泄，一度火灭，一度火灭，一度增油。若不制而纵欲，则是膏火将灭，更去其油。

The present book says: The elderly need to be cautious and restrain their sexual activity for they are weak in blood and qi. They should not indulge themselves in sexual activity irregularly and blindly, just as fire burning and fire being extinguished, fire burning again with addition of lamp oil. Otherwise, they would be perished both in body and essence.

《庄子》曰：嗜欲深者，其天机浅。

Zhuangzi（《庄子》, *Zhuangzi*）, a philosophical work of Taoism in the Warring States period, says: A person who is deeply addicted in desires is endowed with little natural ingenuity and wisdom.

春秋秦医和，视晋侯之疾，曰："是谓近女室，非鬼非食，惑以丧志。"公曰："女不可近乎。"对曰："节之。"

Yi He, a famous physician from Qin State in the Spring and Autumn Period, went to diagnose the disease of the Marquis of Jin and said, "The cause of your disease is sexual overindulgence instead of ghost and diet, and your spirit is misled by it." The Marquis of Jin said, "Is sexual activity not permitted?" He replied, "You need to control your sexual desire."

《玄枢》曰：元气者，肾间动气也。右肾为命门，精神之所舍，爱惜保重，荣卫周流，神气不竭，可与天地同寿。

Xuan Shu（《日月玄枢论》, *The Theory of Alchemy of the Sun and the Moon*）says: The original qi is the dynamic qi between the kidneys. The kidney on the right side is the life-gate where the essence and spirit is stored. If it is cherished well and carefully protected, the nutrient and defensive qi will flow smoothly inside the body and the vitality and spirit will never be exhausted, then the longevity can be achieved.

《元气论》曰：嗜欲之性，固无穷也，以有极之性命，遂无涯之嗜欲，亦自毙之甚矣。

Yuan Qi Lun（《元气论》, *Discussion on the Original Qi*）says: The addiction for desire is infinite while life is limited. It is something like a kind of suicide if one tried to seek pleasure from infinite desires with limited life.

《仙经》云：无劳尔形，无摇尔精，归心静默，可以长生。经颂云：道以精为宝，宝持宜秘密。施人则生人，留己则生己。结婴尚未可，何况空废弃。弃损不觉多，衰老而命坠。

Xian Jing（《仙经》, *The Book of Immortals*）says: Don't overstrain the physique, don't consume the essence too much. One can live a long life if the mind remains at a state of serenity. The Sutra says: The law of nature takes the essence as the most precious thing and it should be supported and maintained secretly. It will benefit others if they know this point and benefit oneself if one knows it. It is not easy for a fetus to take his form, so one should never neglect and damage his life. If a person does not realize the severity of such kind of neglect and damage, he will become aging and lose

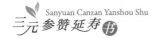

his life.

《仙书》云：阴阳之道，精液为宝。谨而守之，后天不老。

Xian Shu（《仙书》, *The Book of Immortals*）says: The semen is the most precious thing in the law of sexual activity. One will live a long life if it is preserved and valued cautiously.

书云：声色动荡于中，情爱牵缠，心有念，动有着，昼想夜梦，驰逐于无涯之欲，百灵疲役而消散，宅舍无宝而倾颓。

The present book says: If one tries to seek sensual pleasure and emotional involvement, he will be fascinated and directed by this thought in mind and behavior day and night pursuing infinite desires. A man's life may be ended due to this kind of overstrain just like a lark that loses its voice due to tiredness and a house that loses its treasure and falls down.

书云：恣意极情，不知自惜，虚损生也。譬枯朽之木，遇风则折；将溃之岸，值水先颓。苟能爱惜节情，亦得长寿也。

The present book says: If a person indulges in emotions and sexual desires at will without cherishing his own body, deficiency and damage may occur. For example, a withered and rotten tree is easy to be broken when there is wind blowing; a fragile dam is easy to collapse when flood happens. If a person can treasure his body and control his emotions and sexual desire, he can live a long life.

书云：肾阴内属于耳中，膀胱脉出于目眦，目盲所视，耳闭厥聪，斯乃房之为患也。

The present book says: The ear is related with the kidney yin internally and the eye with the bladder by meridian. So blindness and deafness is caused by sexual overindulgence correspondingly.

书云：人寿夭在于樽节，若将息得所，长生不死，恣其情，则命同朝露。

The present book says: The longevity of a person is dependent on the restraint of desires. He may live a long life if the desire is regulated and moderated properly; he may die soon if he indulges in sensual pleasures at will just as the morning dew that disappears without a trace in the blink of an eye.

书云：欲多则损精。人可保者命，可惜者身，可重者精。肝精不固，目眩无光；肺精不交，肌肉消瘦；肾精不固，神气减少；脾精不坚，齿发浮落。若耗散真精不已，疾病随生，死亡随至。

The present book says: The stronger a person's sexual desire is, the easier it is to damage the essence. It is the life that one should preserve, the body that one should cherish, the essence that one should value. If the liver's essence is not consolidated, the eyes will be blurred and dull; if the lung's essence is insufficient, emaciation may occur; if the kidney's essence is not strengthened, one will be dispirited; if the spleen's essence is insufficient, the teeth and hair will fall out. If the vital essence is consumed and damaged

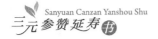

continuously, disease may occur and death may come.

"神仙可惜许歌" 曰：可惜许，可惜许，可惜元阳宫无主。一点既随浓色妒，百神泣送精光去。三尸喜，七魄怒，血贩气衰将何补。尺宅丹田属别人，玉炉丹灶阿谁主。劝世人，休恋色，恋色贪淫有何益？一神去后百神离，百神去后人不知。几度待说说不得，临临下口泄天机。

The Song on Pityful Things by Immortals says: It's a pity! It's a pity! It is a pity that the primordial yang is not preserved well in the kidney. The essence is exhausted little by little due to sexual overindulgence and envy till it is diminished to none eventually with crying and sighing of immortals. The three dead bodies are happy and the seven souls are angry about the despair and hopelessness to tonify the blood and qi. After death, the luxurious house and the vast field will be occupied by others, the jade stove and hearth where the immortality pills are refined have new owners. It is advised that people ought to be far away from sexual overindulgence because it is of no good and benefit. All the thoughts disappear after death and nothing about spirit is left after death. There were times when I wanted to warn people against it but I did not have the opportunity with the fear that the mysteries of nature may be let out.

欲不可强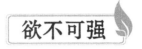

Sexual Activity Kept within One's Capability

《素问》曰："因而强力，肾气乃伤，高骨乃坏。"注云："强力，入房也。强力入房则精耗，精耗则肾伤，肾伤则髓气内枯，腰痛不能俯仰。"

Su Wen（《素问》, *Plain Questions*）says: Over-exertion damages kidney qi and the spine on the lumbar region. The note says: Over-exertion refers to grudging sexual activity. It may consume the essence, damage the kidney and exhaust the marrow, which leads to backache and makes lying flat impossible.

《黄庭经》云：急守精室勿妄泄，闭而宝之可长活。

Huang Ting Jing（《黄庭经》, *The Classic of the Yellow Yard*）says: Do not ejaculate recklessly and preserve the essence cautiously. Cherish and store it well and then one can live a long life.

书云：阴痿不能快欲，强服丹石以助阳，肾水枯竭，心火如焚，五脏干燥，消渴立至。近讽曰：少水不能灭盛火，或为疮疡。

The present book says: If the sexual desire cannot be satisfied due to the

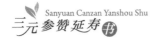
impotence, the taking of elixir pills may cause the depletion of the kidney water, the burning heat of heart fire, the dryness of internal organs and the consumptive thirst eventually. Jin Ne said, "The kidney water cannot put out the heart fire, which may lead to ulcer and sores."

书云：强勉房劳者，成精极、体瘦、尪羸、惊悸、梦泄、遗沥、便浊、阴痿、小腹里急、面黑耳聋。真人曰：养性之道，莫强所不能堪尔。《抱朴子》曰：才不逮，思之，力不胜，强举之，伤也甚矣。强之一字，真戕生伐寿之本。夫饮食所以养生者也，然使醉而强酒，饱而强食，未有不疾而害其身，况欲乎？欲而强，元精去，元神离，元气散，戒之。

The present book says: Overstrain due to sexual activity with difficulty may lead to essence depletion, emaciation, tabid body with arthrocele, fright, nocturnal emission, enuresis, turbid urine, impotence, diarrhea, dark complexion and deafness. The immortal said, "The way to preserve health is not to behave forcefully beyond one's capacity." *Bao Pu Zi*（《抱朴子》, *The Master Who Embraces Simplicity*）says: The intellect can't reach that level, but I force myself too hard to achieve it; the strength is incompetent, but I force myself to lift and the damage may be severe. The word "force" is really the root cause of the destruction of life and the reduction of life expectancy. The normal diet is beneficial for health cultivation. However, if one continues to drink after drunk and eat after full, his health may be damaged by diseases. Is it not the true with the sexual desire? To have sexual activity beyond one's capacity can consume the essence, separate the primordial spirit and dissipate the primordial qi, which should be avoided.

欲有所忌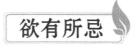

Taboos about Sexual Activity

书云：饱食过，房室劳损，血气流溢，渗入大肠，时便清血，腹痛，病名肠癖。

The present book says: Overeating and overstrain due to sexual activity may lead to the extravasation of blood into the large intestine and cause black feces and abdominal pain, which is named intestinal mass.

书云：大醉入房，气竭肝伤，丈夫则精液衰少，阴痿不起；女子则月事衰微，恶血淹留，生恶疮。

The present book says: The liver may be damaged and qi be exhausted when having sexual activity after being drunk. Man will suffer from decrease in semen and impotence; woman will suffer from malignant sore due to declining menstruation and stasis of extravasated blood.

书云：燃烛行房，终身之忌。

The present book says: Sexual activity with a candle on is a taboo for

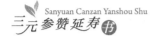

the whole life.

书云：忿怒中尽力房事，精虚气节，发为痈疽。恐惧中入房，阴阳偏虚，发厥、自汗、盗汗，积而成劳。

The present book says: Carbuncle-abscess may occur due to essence deficiency and qi stagnation when having sexual activity in anger. Overstrain may be caused by faint, spontaneous sweating and night sweat due to deficiency of yin and yang when having sexual activity in fear.

书云：远行疲乏入房，为五劳虚损。

The present book says: Exhaustion of the five internal organs and deficiency may be caused by having sexual activity after a long and tiring journey.

书云：月事未绝而交接，生白驳。又冷气入内，身面萎黄，不产。

The present book says: Sexual activity during menstruation may lead to vitiligo, sallow facial complexion and infertility due to the invasion of cold into interior organs.

书云：金疮未瘥而交会，动于血气，令疮败坏。

The present book says: Incised wound may be deteriorated due to blood and qi turbulence when having sexual activity before its recovery.

书云：忍小便入房者，得淋疾，茎中疼痛，面失血色，或致胞转，脐下急痛死。

The present book says: Sexual activity with a full bladder may lead to gonorrhea, penis pain, pale complexion, dysuria with lower abdominal colic and acute pain below the navel.

书云：或新病可而行房，或少年而迷老，世事不能节减，妙药不能频服，因兹致患。岁月将深，直待肉尽骨消，返冤神鬼，故因油尽灯灭，髓竭人亡。添油灯壮，补髓人强，何干鬼老来侵，总是自招其祸。

The present book says: Damage may be caused by sexual activity after newly recovered disease, confusion of the young about the aging, complex and burdensome affairs of life and frequent taking of drugs. With the passing of time, the muscle and bones will be depleted and the acupoints in disorder, which may result in the marrow exhaustion and even death just like the lamp burning itself out. The lamp will not be expired with oil added in time and the body will be vigorous with marrow supplemented often. So the disaster is not caused by external pathogenic factors but by internal factors.

书云：交接输泻，必动三焦，心脾肾也，动则热而欲火炽，因入水，致中焦热郁发黄；下焦气胜，额黑；上焦血走，随瘀热行于大便，黑溏。男女同室而浴者，多病死。

The present book says: The essence purging of sexual activity has impact on the triple energizers, namely the heart, the spleen and the kidney. The sexual desire may produce heat and when encountered water, lead to heat stagnation and yellowish complexion in the middle energizer; the qi

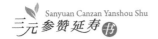
exuberance in the lower energizer may lead to black forehead; the blood extravasation in the upper energizer may flow downward with the heat stagnation to the feces, leading to black loose stool. Those who have sexual activity in bath often suffer from this disorder.

书云：服脑麝入房者，关窍开通，真气走散。重则虚眩，轻则脑泻。

The present book says: Those who have sexual activity after taking musk are open in the joints and orifices, making the genuine qi dissipated. So they often suffer from brain dredging and even dizziness.

《本草》云：多食葫行房，伤肝，面无光。

Ben Cao（《本草》, *Classic of Material Medica*）says: Sexual activity after taking gourds may damage the liver and make the complexion lusterless.

书云：入房汗出中风，为劳风。

The present book says: The wind stroke due to sweating during sexual activity is called wind due to overstrain.

书云：赤目当忌房事，免患内障。

The present book says: Sexual activity should be contraindicated when suffering from pinkeye to avoid cataract.

书云：时病未复，犯者舌出数寸，死。《三国志》子献病已瘥，华佗视脉曰："尚虚未复，勿为劳事，色复即死，死当舌出数寸。"其妻从百里外省之，止宿，夜交接，三日病发，一如佗言。可畏哉。

The present book says: Those who have sexual activity when suffering from seasonal and infectious disease may die with the tongue protruded inches out of the mouth. According to *San Guo Zhi* (《三国志》, *Three Kingdoms*), there was a postal supervisor named Dun Zixian who has just recovered from an infectious disease and went to Hua Tuo for therapeutic advice. After checking his pulse, Hua Tuo said, "You are still weak and not fully recovered. Don't have sexual activity, otherwise you will die with the tongue protruded inches out of the mouth." But he didn't listen and had sexual activity at night when his wife came to visit him from hundreds of miles away. Three days later, he died just as what Hua Tuo said. How scary it is!

欲有所避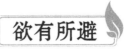

Conditions to Keep off for Sexual Activity

孙真人曰：大寒与大热，且莫贪色欲。

Sun Zhenren（also named Sun Simiao）said, "Don't indulge in sexual desire when it's too cold or too hot."

书云：凡大风、大雨、大雾、雷电霹雳、日月薄蚀、虹霓地动、天地昏冥、日月星辰之下、神庙寺观之中、井灶圊厕之侧、塚墓、尸柩之傍，皆所不可。若犯女，则损人神。若此时受胎，非止百倍损于父母，生子不仁、不孝，多疾损寿。

The present book says: People should neither have sexual activity at the time when there is strong wind, heavy rain, thick fog, lightning and thunder, solar and lunar eclipse, rainbow, earthquake and dusky weather, nor at places where it is under the sun, moon and stars, inside the temples, near the well, hearth and toilet, next to the grave, body and coffin. If they have, the vitality may be damaged, the fetus conceived may be very harmful to their parents, the children born may be heartless, unfilial, sickish and short-lived.

唐·魏征令人勿犯长命及诸神，降日犯淫者，促寿。及《保命诀》所载：

Wei Zheng of the Tang Dynasty warned that people should not violate the same zodiac date as their own, and should not offend Gods by having sexual activity at the days when they descend to the world. Otherwise, their lifespan may be shortened. There is also a record in *Bao Ming Jue*（《保命诀》, *The Secret for Safeguarding the life*）：

朔日减一纪；望日减十年；晦日减一年；初八上弦、二十三下弦，三元减五年；二分、二至、二社，各减四年；庚申甲子本命减二年。正月初三万神都会，十四十六三官降，二月二日万神会，三月初九牛鬼神降，犯者百日中恶。四月初四万佛善化，犯之失音。初八夜盖恶童子降，犯者血死。五月三个五日、六日、七日为九毒日，犯者不过三年。十月初十夜，西天王降，犯之一年死。十一月二十五日，掠剩大夫降，犯之短命。十二月初七夜犯之恶病死；二十日天师相交行道，犯之促寿。每月二十八人神在阴；四月十月阴阳纯用事。已上日辰，犯淫且不可，况婚姻乎？

If people violate the rule and have sexual activity on the new day of the lunar calendar, or the first day of the new year, their lifespan will be reduced by 12 years; on the fifteenth day of the month, their lifespan will be reduced by 10 years; on the last day of the month, their lifespan will be reduced by 1 year; on the 8th and 23rd day of the month, as well as the 15th day of the first month, the 15th day of the seventh month, and the 15th day of the tenth month, their lifespan will be reduced by 5 years; on the Spring Equinox Day,

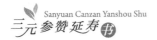
Autumnal Equinox Day, Summer Solstice Day, Winter Solstice Day, Spring Society Day and Autumn Society Day in the 24 solar terms, their lifespan will be reduced by 4 years; in the year of Geng Shen, Jia Zi[1], and animal year, their lifespan will be reduced by 2 years. If people have sexual activity on the third day of the first lunar month when all the Gods meet, on the fourteenth and sixteenth day when the Heavenly God, Earth God and Water God descend, on the second day of the second lunar month when all the Gods meet, and on the ninth day of the third lunar month when monsters and demons descend, they will suffer from bad luck within 100 days. If people violate the rule and have sexual activity on the fourth day of the fourth lunar month when all Buddhist Bodhisattvas hold good-enhancing activities, they will lose their voice; at the night of the eighth day of the first lunar month when the Lad God in charge of good and evil descends, they will die of blood disorder; on the 5th, 15th, 25th, 6th and 7th of the fifth lunar month, they will die within three years; at the night of the tenth day of the tenth lunar month when the Western Heavenly King descends, they will die within a year; on the 25th of the 11th lunar month when the Looter God descends, they will be short-lived; at the night of the seventh day of the twelfth lunar month, they will die of malignant disease; on the twentieth day when Zhang Tianshi performs his magic, they will have a shortened life span. The Man God is in a state of yin on the twenty-eighth day of each month; the pure yang dominates the fourth month and the pure yin the tenth month of the year. In the above mentioned time, no sexual activity should be allowed, let alone get married.

---

① Jia Zi: 60 years on the Lunar calendar is called "Jia Zi", meaning a full cycle.

按《庚申论》曰：古人多尽天数，今人不尽天年，何则？以其罔知避慎，肆情恣色，暗犯禁忌，阴司减其龄算。能及百岁者，几何人哉？蜀王孟昶，纳张丽华于观侧，一夕迅雷电火，张氏殒。道士李若冲，于上元夜，见殿上有朱履衣冠之士，面北而立，廊下罗列罪人，有女子甚苦，白其师唐洞卿。师曰："此张丽华也，昔宠幸于此，亵渎高真所致。"由是观之，天地间禁忌不可犯也。

Geng Shen Lun（《庚申论》, *Discussion on Gengshen*）says: Most of the ancient people lived to the end of their natural lifespan, why can't the contemporary people live to their natural age? It's because their lifespan is shortened due to their ignorance of the precautions, overindulgence in sexual activity and violation of the taboos. How can people live to 100 years old if they behave like this? There was an emperor of Shu state named Meng Chang who took a concubine named Zhang Lihua near a Taoist temple. One night, Zhang Lihua died when there was thunder and lightning. At the night of Lantern Festival, a Taoist named Li Ruochong saw a full dressed dignitary standing in the temple facing the north and a group of sinners lined in the corridor, among which there was a miserable woman. He told this to his master Tang Dongqing and he replied, "This woman is Zhang Lihua and she suffers like this because she blasphemed against the immortals in the temple by having sexual activity with the emperor. Therefore, a conclusion can be drawn that the taboos in the world should never be violated."

嗣续有方

Proper Methods to Conceive

建平孝王妃姬寺，皆丽无子，择良家未笄女入内，又无子。问褚澄曰："求男有道乎？"澄曰："合男女必当其年，男虽十六而精通，必三十而娶；女虽十四而天癸至，必二十而嫁。皆欲阴阳完实，然后交合，合而孕，孕而育，育而子壮强寿。今也不然，此王之所以无子也。"王曰："善。"未再期，生六男。

During the period of Xiao Qi in the Southern Dynasty with the reign title of Jianping, the concubines of King Xiao were beautiful but they could not conceive. More marriageable girls were taken in but still with no baby born. The king asked a famous physician named Chu Cheng, "Is there any method to bear a son?" Chu Cheng answered, "People should have sexual activity in the prime of life. Though men ejaculate at the age of 16, they should marry after the age of 30; though women have menstruation at the age of 14, they should marry after the age of 20. In this case, they would be sexually mature, conceive, and then bear healthy babies. This principle is not followed now and this is the reason for the king to have no sons. The king said, "You are right." Before the coming of the second year, the king had six sons.

书云：丈夫劳伤过度，肾经不暖，精清如水，精冷如冰，精泄，聚而不射，皆令无子。近讷曰：此精气伤败。

The present book says: A man is unable to have babies if their semen is as clear as water, or as cold as ice, or discharging loosely instead of ejaculating properly due to overstrain or coldness of the kidney meridian. Jin Ne said, "This is caused by damage of essence and qi."

书云：女人劳伤气血，或月候愆期，或赤白带下，致阴阳之气不和，又将理失宜，食饮不节，乘风取冷，风冷之气乘其经血，结于子脏，皆令无子。

The present book says: A woman is unable to have babies if there is disharmony between yin and yang, followed by improper regulation and diet, invasion of wind and cold into the meridian and blood and stagnation in the uterus due to damage of qi and blood, delayed menstruation and leukorrhea with reddish discharge.

书云：月候一日至，三日子门开，交则有子，过四日则闭而无子。又经后一日、三日、五日受胎者，皆男；二日、四日、六日受胎者，皆女。过六日胎不成。凌霄花，凡居忌种此，妇人闻其气，不孕。

The present book says: Women are able to conceive if they have sexual activity 3 days after the menstruation period and unable to conceive 4 days

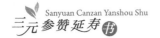

after it because the cervical orifice of uterus will be closed then. There is also a saying that boys may be born if the fetus is formed one day, or three days, or five days after the menstruation period; girls may be born if the fetus is formed two days, or four days, or six days after the menstruation period. Ling Xiaohua（凌霄花, Trumpetcreeper Flower, Flos Campsis）is forbidden to be planted near the living places for its flavor may cause infertility.

妊娠所忌

Taboos during Pregnancy

《产书》云：一月足厥阴肝养血，不可纵欲，疲极筋力，冒触邪风；二月足少阳胆，合于肝，不可惊动；三月手心主，右肾养精，不可纵欲、悲哀、触冒寒冷；四月手少阳三焦合肾，不可劳逸；五月足太阴脾养肉，不可妄思、饥饱、触冒脾湿；六月足阳明胃合脾，不得杂食；七月手太阴肺养皮毛，不可忧郁叫呼；八月手阳明大肠合肺以养气，勿食燥物；九月足少阴肾养骨，不可怀恐、房劳、触冒生冷；十月足太阳膀胱合肾，以太阳为诸阳，主气，使儿脉缕皆成，六腑调畅，与母分气，神气各全，候时而生。所以不说心者，以心为五脏主，如帝王不可有为也。若将理得宜，无伤胎脏。又每月不可针灸其经。如或恶食，但以所思物与之食，必愈。所忌之物，见食物门中。

Chan Shu（《产书》, *The Book of Delivery*）says: In the first month of pregnancy, blood of the fetus is being nourished by the liver channel of foot jueyin and overindulgence in sexual activity is forbidden to avoid the exhaustion of tendons and muscle and the invasion of wind pathogen. In the second month, the gallbladder meridian of foot shaoyang is coordinating with

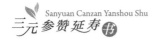
the liver and fright should be avoided. In the third month, the pericardium channel of hand jueyin is in predominance and the essence is being nourished by kidney on the right, so overindulgence in sexual activity, sorrow and cold damage should be forbidden. In the fourth month, the triple-energizer meridian of hand shaoyang is coordinating with the kidney and overstrain should be forbidden. In the fifth month, the spleen meridian of foot taiyin is in predominance and the muscle is growing, so over-thought, hunger and satiation should be forbidden to avoid dampness in the spleen. In the sixth month, the stomach channel of foot yangming is coordinating with the spleen and the diet should be prepared appropriately. In the seventh month, the lung meridian of hand taiyin is in predominance and skin and hair is being nourished, so anxiety, depression, crying and shouting loudly should be forbidden. In the eighth month, the large intestine meridian of hand yangming is coordinating with the lung to supplement qi, so dry food is forbidden. In the ninth month, the kidney channel of foot shaoyin is in predominance and the bones are being formed, so fear, sexual overindulgence and cold damage should be forbidden. In the tenth month, the bladder meridian of foot-taiyang is coordinating with the kidney, which constitutes all the yang of the body and governs qi to shape up the meridians and six fu-organs. At this time the fetus has developed his own spirit and essential qi and is ready to be delivered. The reason that the heart of fetus is not mentioned above is because of its dominating role among the five zang-organs just like the role of monarch. It will not be damaged if cared and regulated properly. Acupuncture is forbidden during all the months of pregnancy and poor appetite can be

improved if the pregnant woman is provided with food she favors. Taboos during pregnancy can be found in the diet category.

《太公胎教》云：母常居静室，多听美言，讲论诗书，陈说礼乐，不听恶言，不视恶事，不起邪念，令生男女，福寿敦厚，忠孝两全。

Tai Gong Tai Jiao（《太公胎教》, *Prenatal Education of Tai Gong*）says: The pregnant women should always live in a quiet house, listen to good words, read and discuss poetry books and talk about rituals and music instead of listening to vicious remarks, watching wrong-doings and thinking of evil ideas. In this case, the babies born will stay honest and sincere, enjoy happiness and longevity, possess loyalty and filial piety.

演山翁云：成胎后，父母不能禁欲，已为不可。又有临产行淫，致其子头戴白被而出，病夭之端也。

Yan Shanweng said, "Sexual activity is supposed unacceptable after the fetus takes shape. Even more serious is the immature death which is mostly caused by sexual activity near the time of labor leading to the delivery of white-semen-covered baby."

婴儿所忌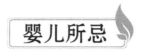

Taboos for Baby

书云：儿未能行，母更有娠，儿饮妊乳，必作魃病，黄瘦骨立，发热，发落。

The present book says: If the mother becomes pregnant again while the baby is breastfeeding and still unable to walk, the baby may suffer from emaciation, boniness, fever and hair-losing due to strange pathogenic factors.

书云：小儿多因缺乳，吃物太早，又母喜嚼食喂之，致生疳病，羸瘦腹大，发竖萎困。

The present book says: The baby may suffer from infantile malnutrition with symptoms of emaciation, swollen abdomen, stiff hair and flaccidity caused by premature taking of food and being fed by chewed food due to hypogalactia.

《养子直诀》云：吃热莫吃冷，吃软莫吃硬，吃少莫吃多。真妙法也。

Yang Zi Zhi Jue（《养子直诀》, *Formulas for Raising Children*）says: For raising children, it is suggested to take hot food instead of cold food, soft food instead of hard food, moderate amount of food instead of excessive amount of food. They are very good tips.

书云：母泪勿堕子目中，令子目破生翳。

The present book says: Mother's tear should not be dropped into the eyes of baby, otherwise slight corneal opacity may occur to the baby.

《琐碎录》云：小儿勿令指月，主生月蚀疮；勿令就瓢及瓶中饮水，令语讷；又衣服不可夜露。

Suo Sui Lu（《琐碎录》, *Record of Trivials*）says: Do not allow the infant to point at the moon, otherwise he may suffer from sores behind his ears. Do not allow the infant to drink water with a gourd ladle or bottle, otherwise he may suffer from stammer. Besides, do not leave children's clothes outside at night.

卷之二
Volume Two

明·钱塘胡文焕（德父）校

Collated by Hu Wenhuan from Qiantang county of Ming Dynasty

地元之寿　起居有常者得之

Prolonging Life by Cultivating Di Yuan

Those Who Lead a Regular Life Can Get It

人之身，仙方以屋子名之。耳、眼、鼻、口其窗牖、门户也；手足肢节其栋梁、榱桷也；毛发体肤其壁瓦、垣墙也。曰气枢、曰血室、曰意舍、曰仓廪玄府、曰泥丸绛宫、曰紫房玉阙、曰十二重楼、曰贲门、曰飞门、曰玄牝等门，盖不一也，而有主之者焉。今夫屋或为暴风疾雨之所飘摇，螫虫蚁蠹之所侵蚀，或又为鼠窃狗偷之所损坏，苟听其自如而不知检，则日积月累，东倾西颓，而不可处矣。盖身者，屋也；心者，居室之主人也。主人能常为之主，则所谓窗户、栋榱、垣壁皆完且固，而地元之寿可得矣。

The human body is compared to a house in effective formulas by immortals. The ears, eyes, nose, and mouth are like the doors and windows of the house; the hands, feet, limbs, joints are like the pillars of the house and the rafters of the roof; the hair and skin are like the wall and tile of the house. In Chinese medicine, the terms like the qi pivot, blood chamber, residence of spirit, granary organ, mansion of sweat, mud pellet (refers to the head) and palace of heart, purple house and jade palace, throat tube, cardia of stomach, mouth, pudendum, are all related with house and they are owned by the master. If the house is swayed by the strong wind and heavy rain, eroded by stinging insects and ants, damaged by rats and dogs, it will become dilapidated and uninhabitable without timely inspect and maintenance. The human body is like the house and the heart is like the master of the house. If the master can take care of the house properly, the windows, pillars, walls will be intact and consolidated, which is true of the human body. In this case, the longevity of the earth can be accomplished.

养生之道

Ways to Preserve Health

老子曰：人生大期，百年为限，节护之者，可至千岁。如膏之小炷与大耳。众人大言，而我小语；众人多烦，而我少记；众人悖暴，而我不怒。不以人事累意，淡然无为，神气自满，以为不死之药。

Lao Zi said, "The normal lifespan of human being is about 100 years, but it can reach 1,000 years if preserved properly. It can be analogized to the small and large wick of the lamp. The others talk loudly, but I speak in a low voice; the others are annoyed a lot, but I forget all the troubles; the others are angry violently, but I keep calm. The secret for immortality is to free the mind from affairs of the world, let things take their own course and keep the vitality vigorous."

庄子曰：能尊生者，虽富贵不以养伤身；虽贫贱不以利累形。今世之人，居高年尊爵者，皆重失之。

Zhuang Zi says: "To preserve health, the rich should not damage the body with excessive use of nourishing methods; the poor should not overstrain the body for seeking benefits. Presently, people with high social status and noble title fail to follow this rule. "

孙真人《铭》曰：怒甚偏伤气，思多太损神，神疲心易役，气弱病相萦。勿使悲欢极，当令饮食均，再三防夜醉，第一戒晨嗔。夜寝鸣云鼓，晨兴漱玉津，妖邪难犯己，精气自全身。若要无诸病，常当节五辛，安神宜悦乐，精气保和纯。寿夭休论命，修行本在人，若能遵此理，平地可朝真。

Ming（《养生铭》, *Epigraph of Health Preservation*）by Sun Simiao says: Excessive anger damages qi, excessive thought damages spirit, exhaustion of spirit damages the heart, qi deficiency causes diseases. The invasion of pathogenic factors can be avoided and the essential qi can be kept sufficient if people stay away from extreme sorrow and joy, keep the diet balanced, restrict from hangover, guard against anger in the morning, cover ears with hands before sleep and swallow saliva in the morning. To keep healthy, one should restrict from taking the five kinds of spicy flavors, calm the mind to be joyous and happy, preserve the essential qi harmonious and purified. The lifespan is not determined by fate but by people themselves and the longevity can be achieved even for ordinary people if they follow this rule.

书云：未闻道者放逸其心，逆于生乐，以精神徇智巧，以忧畏徇得失，以劳苦徇礼节，以身世徇财利。四徇不置，心为之病矣。

The present book says: Those who have no idea about health preservation

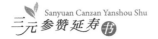
leave their mind unattended and seek pleasure against the natural law. They sacrifice the spirit for craft, sacrifice anxiety and fear for success and failure, sacrifice labor for etiquette, sacrifice life experience for wealth and profit. Disorder may occur to the heart if these sacrifices are dealt with improperly.

陶隐居云：万物惟人灵且贵，百岁光阴如旅寄，自非留意修养中，未免疾苦为身累。

Tao Yinju says, "Human beings are the most intelligent and previous creatures in the nature and their lifespan of 100 years is just as short as a trip. Hardships and sufferings may occur if less importance is attached on the health preservation."

喜 乐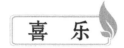

Joy

书云：喜乐无极则伤魄，魄伤则狂，狂者意不存，皮革焦。

The present book says: Excessive joy damages the soul, and then causes mania, and then results in loss of spirit, and finally leads to scorched skin and hair.

书云：喜怒不节，生乃不固。和喜怒以安居处，邪僻不至，长生久视。

The present book says: Excessive joy and anger lead to instability of life. Longevity can be achieved and pathogenic factors can be prevented by moderating joy and anger and securing residence.

书云：喜怒不测，阴气不足，阳气有余，荣卫不行，发为痈疽。

The present book says: Abnormal joy and anger lead to deficiency of yin and excess of yang, which further result in carbuncle-abscess due to the disorder of nutrient qi and defensive qi.

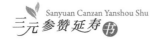
《聚书》云：喜则气和性达，荣卫通行。然大喜伤心，积阳则损，故曰：少喜则神不劳。

Ju Shu（《聚书》, *Collection of Books*）says: The emotion of joy is helpful to harmonize qi and invigorate temperament. However, excessive joy damages the heart and if accumulated it may damage yang of the body. Therefore it is said that moderate joy will benefit the spirit instead of over straining it.

《淮南子》曰：大喜坠阳，大乐气飞扬，恣乐伤魂魄，通于目，损于肝则目暗。

Huai Nan Zi（《淮南子》, *The Huai Nan Zi: A Guide to a Theory and Practice of Government in Early Han China*）says: Excessive rejoicing descends yang qi, excessive joy ascends qi, excessive pleasure-seeking damages soul and spirit. Since this emotion is related with the eyes and the liver, blurred vision may occur due to damage of the liver.

唐柳公度喜摄生，年八十余，步履轻健，或求其术，曰："吾无术，但未常以元气佐喜怒，气海常温耳。"

Liu Gongdu of the Tang Dynasty was good at health preservation. In his 80s, he was still in good health and able to move vigorously. When asked the secret, he said, "I don't have special method and I just have my original qi undamaged by excessive joy and anger, and the Qihai acupoint kept warm."

《东楼法语》曰：心喜则阳气散。是故，抑喜以养阳气。

Dong Lou Fa Yu（《东楼法语》, *Discussion on Health Preservation Methods of Eastern Building*）says: Excessive joy in the heart may consume yang qi. Therefore, it is suggested to moderate joy properly to supplement yang qi.

忿 怒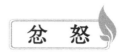

Anger

书云：忿怒则气逆，甚则呕血。少怒则形佚恫恫，忿恨则损寿，怒目久视日月则损明。

The present book says: Rage may cause qi counter-flow even hametemesis. Slight anger may lead to impetuous physique. Resentment may shorten the lifespan. Glaring at the moon and sun for a long time may damage the vision.

书：大怒伤肝，血不荣于筋而气激矣。气激上逆，呕血，飧泄，目暗，使人薄厥。

The present book says: Excessive anger damages the liver and leads to qi surging due to the failure of blood to nourish the tendons. Then the qi counter-flow may result in haematemesis, lienteric diarrhea, blurred vision and even syncope.

书云：切切忿怒，当止之。盛而不止，志为之伤，喜忘前言，腰背隐痛，不可以俯仰屈伸。

The present book says: Severe rage should be stopped timely. Otherwise, it may damage the emotions and lead to poor memory, amnesia, lumbago, backache, inability to lie flat, bend and stretch out the limbs.

书云：多怒则百脉不定。又：多怒则鬓发焦，筋萎，为劳卒，不死，俟五脏传遍终死矣。药力不及，苟能改心易志，可以得生。

The present book says: Frequent anger makes all meridians unstable. It also says: Frequent anger leads to scorched hair on the temples, flaccidity of tendons and even dying state. Eventual death may come when the five zang-organs are damaged by the emotional factor of anger. Though medicinal is not effective in this case, it is still possible to be cured if the mindset can be changed and the emotion can be regulated.

隐居云：道家更有颐生旨，第一令人少嗔恚。

Tao Yinju said, "The first rule of Taoism in health cultivation is to keep from anger and vexation."

书云：当食暴嗔，令人神惊，夜梦飞扬。

The present book says: Great anger during dinner time may lead to fright of spirit and dreaminess at night.

《淮南子》曰：大怒破阴。又：勿恚怒，神不乐。

Huai Nan Zi（《淮南子》, *The Huai Nan Zi: A Guide to a Theory and*

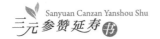
Practice of Government in Early Han China）says: The great rage damages yin. It also says: Vexation and anger may lead to dispiritedness.

《名医叙论》曰：世人不终耆寿，皆由不自爱惜，忿争尽意，聚毒攻神，内伤骨髓，外乏肌肉，正气日衰，邪气日盛，不异举沧波以灭爝火，颓华岳以涓流。

先贤诗曰：怒气剧炎火，焚和徒自伤。触来勿与竞，事过心清凉。

Ming Yi Xu Lun（《名医叙论》, *Famous Doctor's Narrative Theory*）says: The reason that people can not enjoy longevity is that they do not cherish their body health by indulging in anger and fights to accumulate toxin and affect mental health. In this case, the marrow and muscle are damaged internally and externally, which leads to decline of the healthy qi and exuberance of pathogenic factors. It is just like putting out a torch with a sea of water and dam a tiny stream with a mountain of soil.

A poem from the scholar of the past said: Anger intensifies the internal fire and worsens the damage to the body. Do not mind when offended by others and the mind may calm down to a peaceful state afterwards.

悲 哀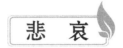

Sorrow

书云：悲哀憔悴，哭泣喘乏，阴阳不交，伤也。故吊死问病，则喜神散。

The present book says: Damage may be caused by imbalance between yin and yang due to sorrow, haggardness, crying and panting. So to offer condolence and visit patients may distract the spirit and depress the mood.

书云：悲哀动中则伤魂，魂伤则狂忘不精，久而阴缩拘挛，两胁痛不举。

The present book says: The spirit may be damaged by internal injury of sorrow, which may lead to mania, amnesia and dispiritedness, even indentation of vulva or penis, pain of hypochondrium and inability to raise arms up.

书云：悲哀太甚，则胞络绝，而阳气内动，发则心下溃，溲数血也。

The present book says: Excessive sorrow stagnates the uterus meridian

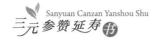
and disturbs yang qi, which may lead to palpitation and bloody urine.

书云：大悲伐性。悲则心系急，肺布叶举，上焦不通，荣卫不舒，热食在中而气消。又云：悲哀则伤志，毛悴色夭，竭绝失生。近讷云：肺出气，因悲而气耗不行，所以心系急而消矣。夫心主志，肾藏志，悲属商，因悲甚则失精，阴缩，因悲而心不乐，水火俱离，神精丧亡矣。

The present book says: The intense sorrow has invasive impact on the temperament by making the heart anxious and the lung stagnated, which may lead to blockage of the upper energizer, dysfunction of the nutrient and defensive qi, and consumption of qi in the middle due to heat pathogen. It also says: The spirit may be damaged by sorrow which can lead to dry hair, pale complexion and loss of vitality. Jin Ne said, "The lung is responsible for respiration and it fails to function well because of the qi exhaustion due to sorrow, so the heart becomes anxious and sluggish. The heart governs the spirit, the kidney stores the spirit, and sorrow pertains to the second tone of Shang among the five tones in TCM. So excessive sorrow may cause the loss of essence and indentation of vulva or penis; excessive sorrow may also cause the separation of water and fire, even the exhaustion of spirit and essence."

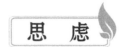

思　虑

Thought

　　黄帝曰：外不劳形于事，内无思想之患，以恬愉为务，以自得为功，形体不弊，精神不散，可寿百数也。

　　Huangdi said, "Physically, they tried not to exhaust their body; mentally, they freed themselves from any anxiety, regarding peace and happiness as the target of their life, and taking self-contentment as the symbol of achievement. As a result, their body was seldom susceptible to decline and their spirit was never subject to exhaustion. That was why they could live over one hundred years."

　　彭祖曰：凡人不可无思，当渐渐除之。人身虚无，但有游气，气息得理，百病不生。又曰：道不在烦，但能不思衣，不思食，不思声色，不思胜负，不思得失，不思荣辱，心不劳，神不极，但尔可得千岁。

　　Pengzu said, "It is natural for human beings to have some thoughts and worries and they will not be harmful if eliminated gradually. No diseases will occur if people can keep the mind tranquil with few desires and regulate

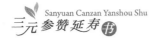
qi to circulate normally." He also said, "The way to preserve health is not complex. A longevity of 1,000 years can be achieved if people do not exhaust their mind and spirit by troubling themselves with the thought of luxurious clothes, improper diet, sensual pleasure, success and failure, loss and gains, honour and disgrace."

庚桑楚曰：全汝形，抱汝生，无使汝思虑营营。

Geng Sangchu said, "Preserve the physique and vitality and keep away from the thought of seeking profits everywhere."

《灵枢》曰：思虑怵惕则伤神，神伤则恐惧自失，破䐃脱肉，毛悴色夭。

Ling Shu（《灵枢》, *Spiritual Pivot*）says: Excessive thought and fear damage the spirit and lead to symptoms of inability to control the emotions, internal exhaustion, emaciation, dry hair and pale complexion.

书云：思虑过度，恐虑无时，郁而生涎，涎与气搏，升而不降，为忧、气、劳、思、食五噎之病。

The present book says: Excessive thought and fear may lead to depression and produce abnormal saliva mixed with the counter flow of qi, which may result in five kinds of choking diseases due to anxiety, anger, overstrain, excessive thought and improper diet.

书云：思虑则心虚，外邪从之。喘而积气在中，时害于食。又云：

思虑伤心，为吐衄，为发焦。

The present book says: Excessive thought may lead to heart deficiency and invasion of exogenous pathogenic factors. Accumulation of qi in the middle due to panting may be harmful to digestion. It also says: Damage of heart due to excessive thought may lead to vomiting, nasal bleeding and anxiety.

书云：谋为过当，食饮不敌，养生之大患也。诸葛亮遣使至司马营，懿不问戎事，但以饮食及事之繁简为问。使曰："诸葛公夙兴夜寐，罚二十以上，皆亲览焉，饮食不数升。"懿曰："孔明食少事烦，其能久乎？"以后果然。

The present book says: Excessive thought without timely supplementation with proper diet is the biggest scourge to health preservation. When Zhuge Liang sent envoy to Sima Yi's war camp, he did not inquire about military affairs but asked about Zhuhe Liang's diet and army management. The envoy answered, "He is hard at work day and night. All the punishments with more than 20 boards need his personal inspection. He ate less than one Sheng each day." Sima Yi said, "He is so busy but eats so little. How can he be sustainable for a long time? This was later confirmed when Zhuge Liang died of overstrain and exhaustion."

张承节云："劳，经言瘵证，有虫，患者相继，诚有是理。只譬如俗谈，不晓事人吉相思病也，与一妇人情密，忽经别离，念念不舍，失察忘餐，便觉形容瘦悴，不偿所愿，竟为沉疴。"

Zhang Chengjie said, "Overstrain is also called consumptive disease in certain classic, which is caused by a kind of harmful worm and is infectious.

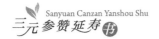

It's said that there was a man falling in love with a woman and suffering from lovesickness. He was reluctant to separate from the woman and missed her so much that he could not sleep or eat anything, which resulted in emaciation and depression and became a severe and lingering disease eventually.

士人有观书忘食。一日，有紫衣人立前曰："公不可久思，思则我死矣。"问其何人？曰："我谷神也。"于是绝思，而食如故。盖思则气结，喉热不散，久而气血俱虚，则疾速至而夭枉也。

There was a scholar who often forgot to eat while reading books. One day, a man in purple stood in front of him and said, "You can't over think for a long time, otherwise I will die." When asked who he was, he said, "I am the Harvest God." So the scholar stopped over-thinking and took dinner as before. Probably excessive thought stagnates qi and results in heat in the throat, which may lead to deficiency of qi and blood over time, quick occurrence of disease, and even death.

忧　愁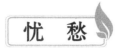

Anxiety

《灵枢》曰：内伤于忧愁则气上逆，上逆则六输不通，温气不行，凝血蕴里而不散，津液涩渗著不去，积遂成矣。

Ling Shu（《灵枢》, *Spiritual Pivot*）says: If there is internal damage due to anxiety and rage, it will drive qi to flow adversely upward. When qi flows adversely upward, the six channels will be obstructed, warm qi cannot flow normally, the blood coagulates and does not disperse, the body fluid cannot flow smoothly, and therefore stagnates in the body. That is how mass is formed.

书云：忧伤肺气而不行。又云：遇事而忧不止，遂成肺劳，胸膈逆满，气从胸达背，隐痛不已。

The present book says: Excessive anxiety damages the lung and leads to stagnation of lung qi. It also says: Continuous anxiety may result in phthisis, counter-flow of qi and fullness in the chest and diaphram, pain in the chest and back due to qi disorder.

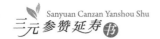

书云：忧愁不解则伤意，恍惚不宁，四肢不耐。

The present book says: Spirit may be damaged if anxiety is not relieved, which may further lead to trance, restlessness and weak limbs.

书云：当食而忧，神为之惊，梦寐不安。

The present book says: Anxiety while taking food may frighten the spirit and lead to restless sleep and dreaminess.

书云：女人忧虑，思想哭泣，令阴阳气结，月水时少时多，内热苦渴，色恶，肌体枯黑。

The present book says: Anxiety and weeping of woman may lead to qi stagnation and bring symptoms like irregular menstruation, thirst due to internal heat, sallow complexion, dry skin and dark body.

书云：深忧重恚，寝息失时，伤也。又云：久泣神悲感，大愁气不通，多愁则心慑。

The present book says: Excessive anxiety and severe vexation may lead to insomnia and cause damage to the body. It also says: Long time of crying leads to grieved spirit, severe anxiety stagnates qi, continuous sorrow frightens the heart.

愁 泣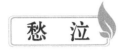

Weeping

《真诰》曰：学生之法，不可泣泪及多唾泄，此皆为漏精损液，使喉脑大痛。是以真人、道士常吐纳咽味，以和六液。

Zhen Gao（《真诰》, *Declarations of the Perfected*）says: The method to have a healthy life is to prevent shedding too much tears and spitting too much saliva, which otherwise may damage the essence and body fluids and cause severe pain of the throat and headache. Therefore, immortals and Taoist priests often practice expiration and inspiration and swallow saliva to harmonize the six kinds of fluids.

又云：哭者亦趣死之音，哀者乃朽骨之大患，恐君子未悟之，相为忧耳。

It also says: Crying sound is what accelerates death and mourning sound is what damages bone. It is pointed out here in case some gentlemen do not realize it and still weep for each other.

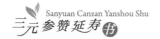
《巢氏病源》曰：哭泣悲来，新哭讫不用即食，久成气病。不可泣泪，使喉涩大渴。愤懑伤神，神通于舌，损心则謇吃。

Chao Shi Bing Yuan（《巢氏病源》, *General Treatise on Causes and Manifestations of All Diseases*）says: Grief often follows crying. Do not have dinner soon after crying, otherwise qi disorder may occur. Do not shed tears too much, otherwise thirst and unsmoothness may occur to the throat. Resentment may damages the spirit and lead to stutter since the spirit is related with the tongue.

惊 恐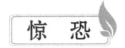

Fright and Fear

书云：因事而有大惊恐，不能自遣，胆气不壮，神魂不安，心虚烦闷，自汗体浮，食饮无味。

The present book says: Great fright and fear, if unrelieved, may lead to weak gallbladder qi, restless spirit, dysphoria and distress of the heart, spontaneous sweating, swollen body and poor appetite.

书云：恐惧不解则精伤，骨酸，痿厥，精时自下，五脏失守，阴虚气不耐。

The present book says: If the fright and fear are not relieved timely, the essence will be damaged, leading to paralyzed bones, spasm, spontaneous seminal emission, disorder of the five internal organs, yin deficiency, weakness and shortness of qi.

书云：惊则身无所倚，神无所归，虑无所定，气乃乱矣。

The present book says: Fright may deprive the body of its dependence,

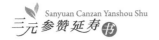
the spirit of its residence, the thought of its settlement and cause qi disorder eventually.

书云：大恐伤肾，恐不除则志伤，恍惚不乐，非长生道。

The present book says: Excessive fear damages the kidney. If unrelieved, it may damage the spirit and cause trance and depression, which is not beneficial for health preservation.

书云：惊恐忧思，内伤脏腑，气逆于上，则吐血也。

The present book says: The emotions of fright, fear, anxiety and thought may damage the internal organs and cause counter-flow of qi and haematemesis.

书云：恐则精却，却则上焦闭，闭则气逆，逆则下焦胀，气乃不行。有妇人累日不产，以坐草太早，恐惧气结而然，遂与紫苏药破气，方得下。

The present book says: Fear may cause the retreat of the essence, then the blockage of the upper energizer, then the qi counter-flow, then the distention of the lower energizer and qi stagnation. Once there was a pregnant woman who was unable to deliver for several days because of early parturiency, fear and qi stagnation. She delivered finally after taking Zisu（紫苏，Perilla Leaf, Folium Perillae）to remove qi stagnation.

书云：临危冒险则魂飞，戏狂禽异兽则神恐。

The present book says: The spirit may be frightened if risking oneself in danger and terrified if teasing wild birds and exotic animals.

《淮南子》曰：大怖生狂。

Huai Nan Zi（《淮南子》, *The Huai Nan Zi: A Guide to a Theory and Practice of Government in Early Han China*）says: Great horror will make people insane.

高逢辰表侄尝游惠山，暮归，遇一巨人醉卧寺门，惊悸不能解，自是便溺一日五六十次。心、小肠受盛府也，因惊而心火散失，心寒肾冷而然，其伤心伤肾之验欤。

Once Gao Fengchen's nephew visited Mountain Hui and met a giant drunk lying at the gate of the temple in the dusk. He was so frightened and terrified that he began to urinate and defecate fifty or sixty times a day. The heart and the small intestine are the organs to receive and store. The heart fire may be dispersed due to the fright, and then lead to kidney cold. This is a case in point to show that fright may damage the heart and the kidney.

有朝贵坐寺中，须臾雷击坐后柱且碎，而神色不动。又有使高丽者，遇风樯折，舟人大恐，其人恬然读书，如在斋阁。苟非所守如此，则其为疾，当何如耶?

There was once an influential official sitting in the temple who remained calm and quiet when the pillars behind him were broken into pieces by thunder. There was also an envoy in a voyage to Korea who continued his reading just like in the study when the mast was broken by strong wind and all the other sailors were terrified. If they did not behave like this, they would have been attacked by diseases. How to deal with the diseases then?

憎 爱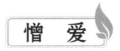

Hatred and Preference

老子曰：甚爱必大费，多藏必厚亡，知足不辱，知止不殆，可以长久。

Lao Zi said: "If you are too partial to something, it will consume a lot of energy and material; if you are too concerned about fame and fortune, then you will also have a big loss. If you know how to be satisfied, you won't be humiliated; and if you know enough is enough, you won't encounter danger and you can have long-term peace."

甚爱色，费精神；甚爱财，遇祸患。所爱者少，所费者多，惟知足知止，则自可不辱而不危也，故可长久。

Indulgence in sexual activity may cause exhaustion of spirit; indulgence in wealth may cause disaster and calamity. To get what one loves needs to pay much higher price. Therefore, those who know how to be satisfied are not humiliated and those who know how to stop in time are not endangered, so that they can enjoy a prolonged life.

书云：憎爱损性伤神。心有所憎，不用深憎，常运心于物平等。心有所爱，不用深爱，如觉偏颇，寻即改正，不然损性伤神。

The present book says: Hatred and preference damages the mind and spirit. Keep the hatred in a moderate degree and try to treat all things equally. Keep the preference in an appropriate degree and regulate it when necessary to avoid damage to the spirit.

书云：多好则专迷不理，多恶则憔悴无欢，乃戕生之斧也。

The present book says: Indulgence in preference may cause irrationality and indulgence in hatred may cause emaciation and unhappiness, which are killers like axe.

《淮南子》曰：好憎者使人心劳，弗疾去则志气日耗，所以不能终其寿。

Huai Nan Zi（《淮南子》, *The Huai Nan Zi: A Guide to a Theory and Practice of Government in Early Han China*）says: Those who tend to have hatred are over-strained in heart. If not relieved timely, it may lead to exhaustion of spirit and shortened longevity.

视 听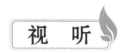

Vision and Hearing

老子曰：五色令人目盲，五音令人耳聋。

Lao Zi said, "The five kinds of colors make people blind and the five kinds of sounds make people deaf."

彭祖曰：淫声哀音，怡心悦耳，以致荒耽之惑，知此可以长生。

Pengzu said, "Sensual and sad music, though joyful and pleasing to the ears, can lead to confusion of indulgence in pleasure. A long lifespan can be assured if this kind of confusion can be avoided."

孔子曰：非礼勿视，非礼勿听。

Confucius said, "Do not look at what is contrary to propriety; do not listen to what is contrary to propriety."

孟子曰：伯夷目不视恶色，耳不听恶声。

Mencius said, "Boyi doesn't look at sensual things and doesn't listen to sensual sounds, either."

孙真人曰：生食五辛，接热食饮，极目远视，夜读注疏，久居烟火，博弈不休，饮酒不已，热餐面食，抄写多年，雕镂细巧，房室不节，泣泪过多，月下观书，夜视星斗，刺头出血多，日没后读书数卷，日月轮看，极目瞻视山川草木，驰骋田猎，冒涉风霜，迎风追兽，日夜不息，皆丧明之由。慎之。

Sun Zhenren said, "The following behaviors should be cautioned and avoided for they may lead to blindness: Take the five kinds of pungent foods while it is uncooked immediately following with hot food; look at the distance as far as one can; take notes and commentaries while reading at night; stay in places with fire and smoke; gamble, play chess and drink ceaselessly; take hot food made of flour; transcribe for many years; carve and engrave exquisitely; indulge in sexual activity; cry and weep too much tears; read under the moonlight; observe the constellation at night; needle with much bleeding; read after the sunset; look at the sun or the moon alternatively; gaze at the landscape, trees and flowers as far as one can; hunt at full gallop; walk in the windy and frosty days; chase after beasts against the wind; take no rest all day and night."

书云：心之神发乎目，久视则伤心；肾之精发乎耳，久听则伤肾。

The present book says: The spirit of heart starts off from the eyes, so long-time of watching impairs the heart; the essence of kidney from the ears, so long-time of hearing impairs the kidney.

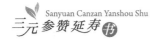
书云：耳耽淫声，目好美色，口嗜滋味，则五脏摇动而不定，血气流荡而不安，精神飞驰而不守，正气既散，邪淫之气乘此生疾。

The present book says: If the ears indulge in sensual sounds, the eyes in woman's beauty and the mouth in tasty foods, the five zang-organs may suffer from unsteadiness, the flowing blood may suffer from restlessness and the spirit may suffer from failure of integration. In this case, diseases may occur with the healthy qi diminished and the pathogenic qi set in.

《叙书》云：久视日月星辰损目，路井莫顾，损寿。故井及水渎勿塞，令人目盲耳聋。玩杀看斗，则气结。

Xu Shu（《叙书》，*The Record of Narration*）says: It may damage the eyes if looking at the sun, the moon and the stars for a long time; it may reduce the lifespan if looking at the well on the roadside. So try to keep the well and the ditch unobstructed, otherwise it may lead to blindness and deafness; try to keep far away from killing and fighting, otherwise qi stagnation may happen.

书云：五色皆损目，惟皂糊屏风可养目力。

The present book says: The five kinds of colors may damage the eyes and the eyesight can be improved by looking at the black folding screen stick with paste.

《淮南子》曰：五色乱目，使目不明；五声哗耳，使耳不聪。又曰：

耳目曷能久熏劳而不息乎？

Huai Nan Zi（《淮南子》, *The Huai NanZi: A Guide to a Theory and Practice of Government in Early Han China*）says: The five kinds of colors disturb the eyes and lead to blurred vision; the five kinds of sounds disturb the ears and lead to loss of hearing. It also says: How can the eyes and ears overwork for a long time without rest?

有年八十余，眸子瞭然，夜读蝇头字。云：别无服药，但自小不食畜兽肝。人以本草羊肝明目而疑之。余曰：羊肝明目，性也。他肝不然，畜兽临宰之时，忿气聚于肝，肝主血，不宜于目明矣。

There was once a person over 80s who had clear eyesight and could read tiny words at night. He said, "I did not take any medicinal and the secret is that I never took domestic or wild animal liver as food since childhood. So it is doubted that whether herbal medicine and sheep liver can improve the eyesight." I said, "It is the property of the sheep liver to improve eyesight, which is not true of the other animals yet. When the other animals are about to be slaughtered, their livers are converged with fright and rage. Since the liver governs the blood, so it is not beneficial to take animal livers for improving the vision."

疑 惑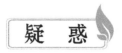

Suspicion

书云：疑惑不已，心无所主，正气不行，外邪干之，失寐忘食，沉沉默默，气血以虚，渐为虚劳。

The present book says: Continuous suspicion leads to the heart losing the function of governing, thus the healthy qi is stagnated and external pathogens invade into the body. Deficiency of blood and qi and consumptive disease may gradually occur with symptoms of insomnia, poor appetite and no desire to speak.

春秋晋侯有疾，秦医和视之，曰："不可为也，疾如蛊。""赵孟曰："何谓蛊？"对曰："淫溺惑乱所生也。于文，皿虫为蛊。在《易》，女惑男，风落山谓之蛊。其卦巽下艮上。巽为长女，为风；艮为少男，为山。少男而悦长女，非匹，故惑。山木得风而落也。"

The emperor of Jin in the Spring and Autumn period was sick, and doctor Yi He of Qin who was invited to treat him said, "The disease is caused by parasitic toxin which cannot be cured." Zhao Meng asked, "What is parasitic toxin?" Yi He answered, "It is caused by indulging in sexual activity and being bewitched by sensual pleasure. From the perspective of word, the Chinese character 'gu' is composed of radical 'min' and 'chong', which basically refer to the insect bred in the utensil for grain. According to *Yi* (《周易》, *The Book of Changes*), parasitic toxin refers to the behavior of women seducing men, just like strong wind blowing trees down from mountain. According to the Eight Diagrams, here the position of Gen is above Xun. Xun refers to the elder woman, which represents the wind; Gen refers to the younger man, which represents the wood. That the younger man attracted by the elder woman is not a perfect match, but a kind of seducing, which is just as the tree blown down by the wind. "

《国史补》云：常疑必为心疾。李蟠常疑遇毒，锁井而饮。心，灵府也，为外物所中，终身不痊。多疑惑，病之本也。昔有饮广客酒者，壁有雕弓，影落杯中，客疑其蛇也，归而疾。作复再饮其地，始知其为弓也，遂愈。又僧入暗室，踏破生茄，疑为物命，念念不释，中夜有扣门索命者，僧约明日荐拔，天明视之，茄也。疑之为害如此。

Guo Shi Bu (《国史补》, *Supplement to the History of the Tang Dynasty*) says: Frequent suspicion may lead to heart diseases. Li Pan of the Tang Dynasty often suspected that the water in his well was poisoned so he locked it. The heart is the residence of spirit. If it is attacked by external pathogens, it will never heal the whole life. Too much suspicion is the root of diseases. Once upon a time, Guang in the Jin Dynasty invited a friend to have a drink in his house. A carved bow was hung on the wall and the shadow of it

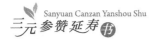
was reflected in the drinking cup just like a snake. The guest thought it was a real snake in his cup and was scared to be sick after returning home. Guang knew the whole story, invited him to drink in his house again and explained to him about the bow. Knowing the truth, his friend recovered soon. And there was another story about a monk stepping on an eggplant when he came into a dark room. He suspected that it was a living creature which was killed by him and was obsessed with it. At midnight, he heard that there seemed to be someone who knocked at his door and asked him to pay for the life. The monk pleaded that he would pray for the dead tomorrow. In the next morning, the monk found that the thing stepped on by him was an eggplant instead of a living thing. How great does suspicion exert influence on people!

谈 笑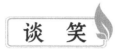

Talking and Laughing

老子曰：塞其兑，闭其门，终身不勤；开其兑，济其事，终身不救。谓目不妄视，口不妄言，终身不勤苦。若目视情欲，又益其事，则没身不可救矣。

Lao Zi says, "Block the orifices of the sensory organs and close the door of desire, one will never be troubled. Open the orifices and allow oneself to indulge, one will be entangled by troubles and never be saved. Namely, do not look around or speak at will, and one will never be troubled. If watching and indulging oneself in sensual pleasure and lust without stop, one will not be saved the whole life."

书云：谈笑以惜精气为本，多笑则肾转腰疼。

The present book says: Too much laughing may cause the twist of kidney and pain in waist, so try to spare the essence and qi when talking and laughing.

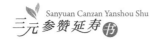

书云：多笑则神伤，神伤则悒悒不乐，恍惚不宁。

The present book says: Too much laughing damages the spirit, which may further lead to depression and trance.

书云：多笑则脏伤，脏伤则脐腹痛，久为气损。

The present book says: Too much laughing damages the zang-organs, which may further cause pain in umbilicus and abdomen, and damage of qi in the long run.

真人云：人若不会将理者，只是多说话。戒多言损气，以全其寿也。

Zhen Ren（Sun Simiao）said, "If people can't express their thoughts rationally, their talk is just a waste of words. Since speaking too much damages qi, people should refrain from it to prolong life."

书云：呼叫过常，辩争问答，冒犯寒暄，恣食咸苦，肺为之病矣。又云：多笑则伤脏，多乐则意溢，多喜则忘错昏乱。

The present book says: The lung may be damaged by frequent shouting, debating and arguing, questioning and answering, offending and greeting, and taking too much salty food. It also says that too much laughing damages the zang-organs, too much joy leads to the mind out of control, and too much delight causes forgetfulness and confusion.

书云：行语令人失气，语多须住乃语。

The present book says: Qi damage may happen if having a talk while walking. So it is supposed to stop walking and then continue the talk.

津　睡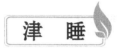

Saliva

真人曰：常习不唾地。盖口中津液，是金浆玉醴，能终日不唾，常含而咽之，令人精气常留，面目有光。

Zhen Ren（Sun Simiao）said, "Do not spit often because the saliva is very precious just like gold liquid and jade wine. Keep the saliva in the mouth all day long and swallow it, which can save the essence and qi and improve the complexion."

书云：养性者，唾不至远，远则精气俱损，久成肺病。手足重，皮毛粗涩，脊痛，咳嗽。故曰远唾不如近唾，近唾不如不唾。

The present book says: Those who are good at health preservation never spit their saliva to a distant place, otherwise it may damage the essence and qi, lead to lung disease in the long run and bring symptoms like heaviness in the limbs, dry and coarse skin and hair, pain in the spine and coughing. Therefore spitting nearer is better than spitting further, and no spitting is better than spitting nearer.

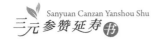

书云：唾者，嗌为醴泉，聚流为华池府，散为津液，降为甘露，溉脏润身，宣通百脉，化养万神，肢节毛发，坚固长春。

The present book says: The saliva is like sweet spring if held by the throat and residence to live in if flowing in the mouth. Saliva, dispersed as fluids and descended as sweet dew, can moisten the zang-organs and the whole body, free the vessels, nourish the spirit, limbs and joints and hair, and strengthen the body and keep one youthful for life.

书云：人骨节中有涎，所以转动滑利。中风则涎上潮，咽喉滚响，以药压下，俾归骨节可也。若吐其涎，时间快意，枯人手足，纵活亦为废人。小儿惊风，亦不可吐涎也。《仙书》云：亥子日不可唾，亡精失气，灭损年命。

The present book says: The sticky fluid in the intersection of bones helps the joints move smoothly. But wind stroke causes the fluid to move upward and sound loudly in the throat. Descend it with medicine to make it return to the joints. If spitting saliva at will, it may cause flaccidity of the limbs and even disability. Saliva should not be spit in the condition of infantile convulsion. *Xian Shu*（《仙书》, *The Book by Immortals*）says: Spitting is forbidden on the day of Hai and Zi, since it can exhaust the essence and qi and shorten the lifespan.

有人喜唾，液干而体枯，遇至人教以回津之法，久而体复润。盖人身以滋液为本，在皮为汗，在肉为血，在肾为精，在口为津，伏脾为痰，在眼为泪。曰汗、曰血、曰泪、曰精，出则皆不可回，为津唾则独可回，回则生意又续矣。滋液者，吾身之宝。《金丹诀》曰：宝聚则为富家翁，宝散则为孤贫客。

There was someone who often spit and was exhausted in body fluid with dry body. His body became moist again when a saint encountered taught him the method to restore the body fluid. The body fluid is the essence of human's body, manifested as sweat in the skin, blood in the flesh, essence in the kidney, saliva in the mouth, phlegm hidden in the spleen, and tears in the eyes. Once discharged, the sweat, blood, tears or essence cannot be restored except saliva. The restoring of saliva can bring the life back. So body fluid is the precious treasure of the body. *Jin Dan Jue*（《金丹诀》, *Golden Elixir Formmula*）says: The gathering of treasure makes one rich, and the losing of it makes one lonely and poor.

起 居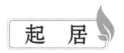

Daily Life

广成子曰：无劳尔形，无摇尔精，乃可以长生。所谓无劳者，非若饱食坐卧，兀然不动，使经络不通，血气凝滞。但不必提重执轻，吃吃终日，无致精力疲极，则妙矣。

Guang Chengzi said, "Do not overstrain the body or exhaust the essence, then the longevity can be achieved." No overstrain does not refer to sitting or lying with satiation doing nothing, which may lead to blockage of meridians and stagnation of blood and qi. It is regarded beneficial to health if heavy load, motionlessness all day and exhaustion of essence can be avoided.

庄周曰：人有畏形恶迹而走，举足愈数而迹愈多，走愈疾而影不随，是自以为尚迟，疾走不休，绝力而死。不知处阴以休影，处静以息迹，遇亦甚矣。

Zhuang Zi said, "One may keep running for fear of his own shadow and footprints left. Whereas more footprints are left when stepping much quickly and the shadow always follows closely however fast the running is. One may keep running till death due to exhaustion if assuming the reason being the running speed not fast enough. How innocent it is without knowing to cover the shadow under the shade or stay still to hide the footprints!"

书云：勇于敢则杀，勇于不敢则活。盖敢于有为即杀身，不敢有为则活其身也。

The present book says: To be bold in daily life brings danger to life and to avoid boldness secures life. The reason is that involving in bold affairs risks life, avoiding bold affairs saves life.

书云：起居不节，用力过度，则络脉伤，伤阳则衄，伤阴则下。

The present book says: Irregular and over-strained lifestyle damages the collaterals. It may cause nose-bleeding if yang collateral is damaged and diarrhea if yin collateral is damaged.

书云：起居不时，食饮不节者，阴受之而入五脏，填满拍塞，为飱泄，为肠澼。贼风虚邪者，阳受之而入六腑，身热不得卧，上为喘呼。

The present book says: Irregular life pattern and imbalanced diet may cause yin damage and affect the five zang-organs, leading to fullness, stagnation, diarrhea and intestinal mass. Exogenous pathogenic factors may cause yang damage and affect the six fu-organs, leading to inability to lie down due to body heat and asthma.

书云：精者，神之本。气者，神之主。形者，气之宅。神大用则歇，精大用则竭，气大劳则绝。

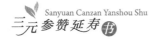
The present book says: Essence is the basis of spirit, qi is the governor of spirit and body physique is the residence of spirit. Excessive consumption of spirit leads to sluggishness, excessive consumption of essence leads to exhaustion, and excessive consumption of qi leads to death.

书云：清旦常言好事，勿恶言。闻恶事，即向所来方唾之三遍，吉。又勿嗔怒，勿叱咤咄呼，勿嗟叹，勿唱奈何，名曰请祸。

The present book says: Talk about good things in the morning instead of bad things. It is auspicious to spit three times toward the direction of the source of bad news. Moreover, it is not supposed to get angry, scold and shout angrily, sigh or exclaim unreasonably, all of which can cause troubles and disasters.

书云：早起以左右手摩肾，次摩脚心，则无脚气诸疾。以热气摩面，则令人悦色，以手背揉眼，则明目。

The present book says: In the morning, massage the kidney with hands first and then the soles to keep away from diseases like beriberi. Massage the face with warm palms to improve the complexion and massage the eyes with dorsum of hands to improve the eyesight.

煨生姜早晨含少许，生胃气，辟山瘴邪气。

Stew fresh ginger and keep a small amount of it in the mouth in the morning to generate stomach qi and eliminate miasmic and pathogenic qi.

早起先以左足下床，则一日平宁。

In the morning, get up and step down on the ground with the left foot first, which can ensure the whole day peaceful.

每日下床，先左脚，念"乾元亨利贞"；下右足，念"日日保长生"。如此各念三遍，则终日吉。

In the morning, get up and step on the ground with the left foot first and right foot second, uttering auspicious words of "Qian Yuan Heng Li Zhen" in Chinese（Refers to four virtues of the Qian Diagram from Book of changes, meaning good luck）and "Long life blessed" respectively for three times to pray for health and longevity, which brings good luck all day.

晨兴以钟乳粉入白粥中，拌和食之，极益人。

Mix the powder of stalactite into porridge and take it in the morning, which benefits health greatly.

早起不可用刷牙子，恐根浮，兼牙疏，易损极，久之患牙疼。盖刷牙子皆是马尾为之，极有所损。今时出牙者，尽有马尾灰，盖马尾能腐齿根。

Do not use the brush to clean the teeth in the morning for fear of gingival loosening and sparse teeth, which leads to toothache in the long run. The reason is that toothbrush is usually made of horsetail hair, which damages teeth a lot. Presently the newly sprouted teeth are in the color of grey horse-tail due to the function of the horse tail to decay teeth.

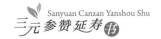
书云：早起向东坐，以两手相摩令热，以手摩额上至顶上，满二九，正名曰存泥丸。

The present book says: In the morning, get up and sit toward east, rub the palms till they are warm and massage the region from the forehead to the top of the head for eighteen times, which is called Cun Ni Wan in Chinese, a term from Qigong meaning invigorating the brain with massage practice.

清旦初起，以两手又两耳，极上下，之二七止，令人不聋。次缩鼻闭气，右手从头上引左耳二七止，次引两发鬓，举之，令人血气流通，头不白。又摩手令热，以摩身体，从上至下，名干浴，令人胜风寒时气，寒热头疼，百病皆除之。

When getting up in the morning, rub the ears from top to bottom with hands for fourteen times, which improves the hearing. Then contract the nostrils to hold the breath, pull the left ear with the right hand for fourteen times, then lift the hair on the temples, which can improve the circulation of blood and qi, and keep the hair black. Finally, rub the palms till they are warm and massage the body from top to bottom, which is called "Gan Yu" in Chinese, meaning bathing without water. This may help to resist the wind-cold and seasonal epidemic, treat headache due to cold-heat and other diseases.

凡人旦起，常言善事，天与之福。

Whenever one gets up in the morning, talk about good things and then one will be blessed with good luck.

夜起坐以手攀脚底，则无筋转之疾。

Reach and touch the soles of the feet with the hands when sitting up at night, which helps to stay away from spasm.

行 立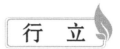

Walking and Standing

书云：久行伤筋，劳于肝；久立伤骨，损于肾。

The present book says: Long time of walking hurts the sinews, which overstrains the liver; long time of standing hurts the bones, which damages the kidney

《养生》云：行不疾步，立不至疲，立勿背日。

Yang Sheng（《养生》, *Health Preservation*）says: Do not walk at a fast speed, do not stand wearily, do not stand against the sun.

书云：奔走及走马，大动其气，气逆于膈未散而又饮水，水搏于气，为上逆。

The present book says: Running at the speed of a galloping horse disturbs qi and causes counter-flow and stagnation of qi in the diaphram, which is worsened with the drinking of water at this time and leads to entanglement of water and qi and reverse flow of qi eventually.

书云：水有沙虱处勿浴勿渡，当随牛马急渡之，不伤人。水中又有弩，射人影即死。以物打水，令弩散，急渡，吉。

The present book says: Do not cross or bathe in the river with chigger mite. In this case, it is safe to cross the river together with cows or horses at a fast speed. There are also noxious insects called Shui Nu in the river, which can shoot people dead with sand. Thus before crossing the river, throw something toward these insects and scatter them, then crosse the river at a fast speed, which can be regarded as a good method.

书云：行汗勿跂床悬脚，久成血痹，足痛腰疼。

The present book says: Do not stand on tip toe for long time with foot suspended when there is sweat, which may lead to blood impediment, pain in the foot and the waist.

真人曰：夜行常啄齿，杀鬼邪。又：疾行损筋。行不得令人失气。又：行及乘马，不用回顾，则神去。

Zhen Ren（Sun Simiao）said, "Knock the teeth often to dispel pathogenic factors when walking outside at night." He also said, "Walking too fast damages the sinew. Prevent the loss of qi when walking." He also said, "Do not look back when walking or riding a horse, otherwise the spirit may be lost."

凡欲行来，常存魁罡在头上，所向皆吉。

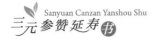
When planning to set out on a journey, walk under the stars of Doukui and Tiangang, which may bring good luck.

行不多言，恐神散而损气。

Do not talk much when walking, otherwise it may lead to distraction of spirit and damage of qi.

夜行常琢齿，琢齿亦无限数也，煞鬼邪。鬼邪畏琢齿声，是故不敢犯人。

Knock on the teeth as much as possible to dispel evil and pathogenic factors when walking outside at night. They are afraid of the sound of knocking teeth, so they dare not attack people.

夜行及冥卧心中恐者，存日月还入于明堂中，须臾百邪自灭，山居恒尔此为佳。

If you are scared when walking at night or lying in meditation, keep the image of the sun and the moon around the nose and then all the pathogens may disappear, which is especially effective for those who live in the mountain.

夜归，左手或右手以中指书手心，作"我是鬼"三字，再握固则不恐惧。

When returning home at night, use the middle finger to scribble "I am the ghost" in the palm, clench the fist and then the fear disappears.

沈存中《笔谈》：草间有黄花蜘蛛，名天蛇。遭其螫仍濡露，则病如癞，通身溃烂，露涉者慎之。

Bi Tan（《笔谈》, *Brush Talks from Dream Brook*）by Shen Cunzhong says: The spider with yellow pattern in the grass is called Tianshe. If stung by it and run into the dew, one may suffer from scabies and fester of the whole body, thus one must be cautious when crossing the grass with dew.

书云：大雾不宜远行，行宜饮少酒，以御雾瘴。昔有三人早行，一食粥而病，一空腹而死，一饮酒而健。酒能壮气，辟雾瘴也。

The present book says: Do not have a long journey in the dense fog. If necessary, one should take a small amount of alcohol to resist the fog miasma. Once there were three persons who started a journey in the morning. The one who took porridge during breakfast was sick, the one who took nothing died, while the one who drank alcohol was as healthy as before. The reason is that alcohol could strengthen qi and evade miasma.

坐 卧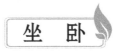

Sitting and Lying

书云：久坐伤肉，久卧伤气，坐勿背日，勿当风湿成劳。坐卧于塚墓之傍，精神自散。

The present book says: Long time of sitting damages the muscle and long time of lying damages qi. Do not sit with the back against the sun and do not sit facing the wind or near the dampness. Sitting or lying near the tomb causes the disperse of the spirit.

书云：卧出而风吹之，血凝于肤为痹，凝脉为血行不利，凝于足为厥。

The present book says: When blown by wind after lying, one may suffer from flaccidity if blood stagnates in the skin, unsmooth circulation of blood if it stagnates in the vessel, syncope if blood stagnates in the feet.

书云：灯烛而卧，神魂不安。卧宜侧身屈膝，不损心气。觉宜舒展，精神不散。舒卧招邪魅。孔子云：寝不尸。

The present book says: Lying with the candle on may disturb the spirit. It is advised to lie on the side with the knees bent to protect the qi of heart. Stretch and relax the feet in sleep to help keep the spirit integrated. Lying in a stretched posture provokes pathogens. Confucius said, "Don't lie with the limbs stretching stiffly in sleep."

书云：寝不得言语。五脏如悬磬，不悬不可发声。孔子曰：寝不言。

The present book says: Do not talk when sleeping. The five-zang organs are like the hanging chime stone, which can produce sound only in the hanging position. Confucius said, "Do not talk when sleeping."

书云：卧不可戏将笔墨画其面，魂不归体。

The present book says: Do not play with painting on the face when sleeping, which may lead to the separation of the spirit with the body.

书云：卧勿以脚悬踏高处，久成肾水，损房足冷。

The present book says: Do not hang the feet high when lying, which may gradually cause fluid stagnation in the kidney, sexual impotence and cold feet.

书云：卧魇魂魄外游，为邪所执，宜暗唤，忌以火照，照则神魂入，乃至死于灯前。魇者本由明出，不忌火，并不宜近唤及急唤，亦喜失神魂也。

The present book says: When one is haunted by nightmare with spirit

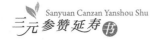
wandering out and constrained by pathogenic factors, he should be called awake in the dark instead of the brightness lighted with lamp to avoid the failure of the spirit to return back to the body and even death before the lamp. Nightmare that comes out of the bright places is not afraid of fire, thus it is inappropriate to call one awake nearby or in a hurry, which may lead to the loss of the spirit.

书云：卧处头边勿安火炉，日久引火气，头重目赤鼻干，发脑痈疮疖。

The present book says: Do not install the stove near the place which is close to the head in the bedroom, which may cause internal heat in the long run, manifested as heavy head, red eyes, dry nose, abscess and sores.

书云：卧习闭口，气不失，邪不入。若张口，久成消渴，无血色。又夜卧勿覆头，得长寿。濯足而卧，四肢无冷病。又醉卧当风，使人发瘖。醉卧黍穰中，发疮，患大风眉堕。又雷鸣时，仰卧星月下，裸卧当风中，醉卧以人扇之，皆不可也。

The present book says: Habituate oneself to sleeping with mouth closed, then there will be no danger of qi loss and invasion of pathogens. Consumptive thirst and pale complexion may occur if keeping the mouth open when sleeping. Do not cover the head with quilt at night, then longevity can be achieved. Wash the feet before sleep, then the limbs will not suffer from cold. Dumbness may occur if one is drunk and invaded by wind pathogen in sleep. Sores and eyebrow shedding may occur if one is drunk and sleeps in the millet stalks. It is forbidden to lie on one's back outside when thundering, or to lie naked facing the wind, or to lie drunk with other people fanning nearby.

隐居云：卧处须当傍虚歇，烘烘衣衾常损人。

Yin Ju（Tao Hongjing）said, "Watch out for the empty space nearby in the bedroom, and the clothes and quilts warmed by fire are harmful to health."

书云：饱食即卧，久成气病，腰痛，百疴不消，成积聚。

The present book says: Sleep with full stomach may cause disorder of qi in the long run, pain in the waist, and various diseases that are hard to cure.

书云：汗出不可露卧及浴，使人身振，寒热风疹。

The present book says: Do not sleep or bathe outdoors when perspiring, which may cause trembling and rubella due to chills and fever.

《西山记》：坐卧于塚墓之间，精神自散。枯木大树之下不可息，防阴气触人阳神。

Xi Shan Ji（《西山记》, West Hill）says: Sitting or lying near the tombs may damage the spirit. Do not rest under the dead and huge trees in case that the yang spirit might be hurt by yin qi.

孙真人曰：坐卧莫当风，频于暖处浴。

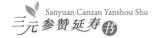
Sun Zhenren（Sun Simiao）said, "Do not sit and sleep facing the wind and bathe in the warm place often."

书云：坐卧处有隙风急避之，尤不宜体虚年老之人。昔有人三代不寿，问彭祖。祖观其寝处，果有一穴，当其脑户，令塞之，遂得寿。盖隙风入耳吹脑，则阳气散。头者，诸阳所聚，以主生也。

The present book says: Keep away from the wind through the openings in the living room, especially for those who are elder and weak. In the past there was a person with three generations of ancestors short-lived, so he came to ask Peng Zu about the reason. Peng Zu examined carefully the place where they slept and found that there was indeed a loophole facing the position of their head when sleeping. The hole was sealed well and then the family could live a long life. The reason is that the wind blowing in through the hole causes disperse of yang qi. The head is the place where yang qi gathers and is the organ that governs vitality.

沐浴洗面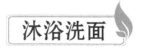

Bathing and Washing Face

书云：频沐者，气壅于脑，滞于中，令形瘦体重，久而经络不通畅。

The present book says: Those who bathe frequently will suffer from qi stagnation in the brain and the middle, which may lead to emaciation, heavy weight and blocked meridians in the long run.

书云：饱食沐发，冷水洗头，饮水沐头，热泔洗头，冷水濯足，皆令人头风。

The present book says: Head wind can be caused by washing hair with full stomach, washing hair with cold water, washing head after drinking water, washing hair with hot rice-washing water and washing feet with cold water.

书云：新沐发勿令当风，勿湿萦髻，勿湿头卧，令人头风、眩闷及生白屑、发秃、面黑、齿痛、耳聋。

The present book says: Do not put the newly-washed hair facing the

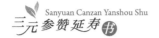
wind, do not wet the bun and do not sleep with wet hair, which may cause recurrent headache, dizziness, dandruff, baldness, dark complexion, toothache and deafness.

书云：女人月事来不可洗头，或因感疾，终不可治。

The present book says: Do not wash hair during menstruation, which may cause exogenous diseases that can not be cured.

书云：沐浴渍水而卧，积气在小腹与阴，成肾痹。

The present book says: To sleep with wet body after bathing may lead to qi stagnation in the abdomen and pudendum, and finally kidney impediment.

书云：炊汤经宿洗体成癣，洗面无光，作甑哇疮。

The present book says: To bathe in the overnight rice-water may cause dermatomycosis. To wash face with it may lead to dark complexion and sores like the surface of the earthen utensil for steaming rice.

书云：频浴者，血凝而气散，体虽泽而气自损，故有痈、疽、疮、疖之疾者，气不胜血，神不胜形也。

The present book says: Those who bathe frequently, though moist and smooth in skin, may suffer from blood stagnation and qi damage, leading to symptoms like carbuncle, abscess, sores and furuncle. The reason is that their blood is not dominated by qi and their body is not dominated by spirit.

书云：时病新愈，冷水洗浴，损心胞。

The present book says: Bathing with cold water after newly recovering from seasonal diseases damages the pericardium.

书云：盛暑冲热，冷水洗手，尚令五脏干枯，况沐浴乎？

The present book says: Washing hands with cold water even in the extreme heat of midsummer can cause disorders of the five-zang organs, let alone bathing.

书云：因汗入水，即成骨痹。

The present book says: Bathing with sweat leads to bone impediment.

昔有名医将入蜀，见负薪者，猛汗河浴。医曰：此人必死。随而救之。其人入店中，取大蒜细切，热面浇之，食之汗出如雨。医曰："贫下人且知药，况富贵乎？"遂不入蜀。

In the past, there was a famous doctor who planned to go to Sichuan. On his journey he saw a person who shouldered the firewood and sweated a lot bathing in the river. The doctor said, "This man is bound to die." Then the doctor followed him and was prepared to save him. He saw the person entered an eatery, asked for chopped garlic, poured it on hot noodles, then ate the noodles and sweated like rain. The doctor said, "Even the poor knows how to treat diseases and keep healthy, not to mention the rich." So he changed his mind and didn't enter Sichuan.

书云：远行触热，逢河勿洗面，生乌𭖊。

The present book says: Do not wash face in the river when travelling afar in a extremely hot weather, which may lead to dark and dry skin.

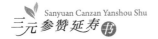

《闲览》云：目疾切忌浴，令人目盲。

Xian Lan（《闲览》, *Leisurely Reading*）says: Do not bathe when suffering from eye diseases, which may lead to blindness.

白彦良壮岁，常患赤目。道人曰：但能不沐头，则不病此。彦良记之，七十余更无眼疾。

When Bai Yanliang was in the prime of his life, he often suffered from red eyes. A Taoist told him, "Do not wash your head and then you will not suffer from the disease again." Bai Yanliang kept that in mind and no longer suffered from eye diseases till seventies.

栉 发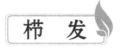

Hair Combing

真人曰：发多栉，去风明目，不死之道。曰：头发梳百度。

Zhen Ren（Sun Simiao）said, "Combing hair often can expel wind, brighten the eyes and prolong lifespan." He also said, "Comb hair for one hundred times each day."

陶隐居云：饱则人浴饥则梳，梳多浴少益心目。

Tao Yinju says, "Take bath when the stomach is full and comb hair when hungry. Combing more and bathing less is beneficial to the heart and eyes."

故道家晨梳，常以百二十为数。

Thus the Taoist usually combs the hair for at least 120 times in the morning.

真人曰：发宜多栉，手宜在面，齿宜数叩，精宜常咽，气宜精炼。

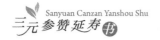
此五者，所谓子欲不终，修昆仑耳。

Zhen Ren（Sun Simiao）said, "It is beneficial to comb the hair frequently, massage the face with the hands often, knock the teeth frequently, swallow the saliva often and practice qi inhalation and exhalation meticulously. These five methods can help to prolong lifespan and are termed Xiu Kun Lun in Chinese, meaning a Taoism method to practice Qigong for health preservation."

《安乐诗》云：发是血之余，一日一次梳，通血脉，散风湿。

An Le Shi（《安乐诗》, *Poetry of Peace and Happiness*）says: The hair originates from blood and is nourished by blood. Thus combing the hair once a day can keep the blood circulate freely and expel wind and dampness.

《琐碎录》云：乱发藏卧房壁中，久招不祥。又云：勿令发覆面，不祥。头发不可在鱼鲊中，食之杀人。

Suo Sui Lu（《琐碎录》, *Record of Trivials*）says: The messy hair put in the cabinet of the bedroom for a long time may bring inauspiciousness. It also says: Covering the face with hair is inauspicious. Do not put hair in the salted fish, which may kill people if taken as food.

《本草》云：收自己乱头发，洗净，干，每一两入椒五十粒，泥固封，入炉，大火一煅，如黑糟，细研，酒服一钱匕，髭发长黑。

Ben Cao（《本草》, *Classic of Materia Medica*）says: Collect the hairs lost, wash and dry them, mix one Liang of hair with fifty grains of pricklyash peel, seal it with mud and put into stove to burn till it turns into black ash, grind it into powder. Take one Qianbi（Refers to metal coin in ancient times, here the weight of a metal coin）together with wine each time, which can keep the hair shiny and black.

刘安君烧自己发，合头垢等分，合服如大豆许三丸，名曰还精。令头不白，服气积义。

It is recorded that Liu Anjun burned his own hair and mix it with dirt on his head. He made the mixture into pills as big as beans and took three each time, which is called "essence recovery". It can help to keep the hair black and benefit the essence and qi.

刘根曰：取七岁男齿女发，与己颈垢合烧，服之，一岁则不知老，常为之，使老有少容也。

Liu Gen said, "Prepare the teeth of a seven-year-old boy and the hair of a seven-year-old girl, burn them together with dirt on the neck and take it. Then one will remain the same without aging after a year. Take it often and the elder may become younger than before."

书云：凡梳头发及爪皆埋之，勿投水火，正尔抛掷。一则敬父母之遗体，二则有鸟，曰鹄鹕，夜入人家，取其爪发，则伤魂。

The present book says: The hair fallen out and the nail cut off should be covered with earth instead of putting into water or fire. For one reason, this can show respect for the parents who give us life; for another reason, if the

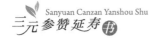
hair and nail are taken away by a kind of bird called bulbul at night, it may damage the spirit.

书云：发落诸饮食中，食之成瘕。

The present book says: Abdominal mass may occur if taking the food with fallen hair in.

宋明帝宫人腰痛引心，发则气绝。徐文伯曰："发瘕也。"以油灌之，吐物长二尺，头已成蛇，悬柱上水沥尽，惟余一发。唐·甄立言为太常，昔有病人心腹满烦弥瘝，诊曰："误食发而然。"令饵雄黄，吐一蛇，如拇指大，无目。烧之，有发气，若头尾全，误食必然。

An imperial secretary of Emperor Ming in the Song Dynasty suffered from sharp pain in the waist and even felt dying when it broke out. Xu Wenbo said, "This is because of the movable abdominal mass in the abdomen." He asked the secretary to drink much oil to induce vomiting and something two feet long like a snake was spit out, which became a hair finally after being hung on a post to drain the water. Zhen Liyan in the Tang Dynasty was a subordinate of Taichang. Once there was a patient who suffered from vexation and fullness in the heart and abdomen came for treatment. Zhen diagnosed him and said, "You ate the hair by mistake." Zhen asked the patient to take realgar as bait and the patient spit out a snake without eyes in the size of a thumb. After burning, it has the smell of hair. So it is the hair taken by mistake that caused the disease if the head and tail of the snake are complete.

大小腑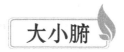

Urination and Defecation

书云：忍尿不便，成五淋，膝冷成痹。忍大便成五痔。

The present book says: Suppression of urination may lead to five kinds of stranguries and impediment due to cold knees. Suppression of defecation may lead to five kinds of hemorrhoids.

书云：弩小便，足膝冷；呼气，弩大便，腰痛目涩。

The present book says: Excessive force during urination leads to cold feet and knees, and excessive force and expiration during defecation leads to lumbago and dry eyes.

书云：或饮食，或走马，或疾走，或为寒热所迫，令胞转，脐下痛，胞屈辟不小便，致死。

The present book says: Improper diet, horse riding, running, or the invasion of cold and heat may lead to dysuria with lower abdominal colic, pain below the navel, difficulty of urination, which may lead to death

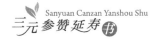
eventually.

《琐碎录》云：夜间小便时，仰面开眼，至老眼不昏。又：丈夫饥欲坐小便，若饱则立小便，慎之无病。

Suo Sui Lu（《琐碎录》，*Record of Trivials*）says: Keep face up and eyes open when urinating at night, then one will not suffer from blurred vision till old. It also says: Men should be cautious and sit to urinate when hungry and stand to urinate when full, which can prevent diseases.

又云：不可对正北溺，及对三光便溺，及向西北，并损人年寿。

It also says: Do not urinate to the direction of due north, or facing the sun, moon and stars, or to the northwest, which may shorten the lifespan.

书云：凡人求道受戒，勿犯五逆，有犯者凶。大小便向南一逆，向北二逆，向日三逆，向月四逆，仰视天及星辰五逆。

The present book says: To pursue the morality and be initiated into monkhood or nunhood, one ought not break the five kinds of rebellious acts, otherwise disaster may occur. The first act is to urinate or defecate toward the south, the second one is to urinate or defecate toward the north, the third one is to urinate or defecate toward the sun, the fourth one is to urinate or defecate toward the moon, the fifth one is to urinate or defecate toward the star with face up.

书云：大小二事，勿强关抑忍，又勿失度，或涩，或滑，皆伤气害生，为祸甚速。

The present book says: Urination and defecation should not be suppressed or purged excessively. The unsmoothness and diarrhea of the urination and defecation may damage qi and vitality of the body quickly.

刘惟简至乾宁军，有人献金花丸，以缩小便，药犯砒蜡，服三日，小便极少。至羁州，肢体通肿。盖被闭却水道，水溢妄行。不遇卢昶，几为所误。盖水泉不止者，膀胱不藏也，宜服暖剂以摄水，可强止之耶?

Once Liu Weijian went to command Qianning's army. Someone presented him with Golden Flower pills to treat frequent urination, which is incompatible with arsenic. After taking it for three days, he urinated little. When marching to Jizhou, his body swelled. The reason was that the channel for urination was blocked and the urine could not be discharged timely and overflowed around the body. If not for doctor Lu Chang, the opportunity of treatment might be delayed. For those who urinate frequently, the reason is that the bladder does not function well in securing and containing urine. In this case, medicinals with warming function should be taken to regulate the water instead of stopping it forcibly.

衣著汗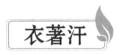

Clothing

书云：春冰未泮，衣欲下厚上薄，养阳收阴，继世长生。

The present book says: When the ice has not melted in spring, the principle of wearing thick clothes at the bottom and thin clothes at the top should be followed to nourish yang qi and restrain yin qi for the purpose of preserving health and prolonging lifespan.

书云：春天不可薄衣，伤寒、霍乱、食不消、头痛。

The present book says: It is not suggested to wear thin clothes in spring, otherwise it may cause cold damage, cholera, indigestion and headache.

书云：冬时绵衣、毡褥之类，急寒急着，急换急脱。

The present book says: Cotton padded clothes, blankets and mattress in winter should be put on and changed in time when the weather turns cold suddenly, and then be taken off and changed when the weather turns warm suddenly.

陶隐居云：绵衣不用顿加添，稍暖又宜时暂脱。

Tao Yinju said, "When it is cold, do not add clothes immediately; when it is warm, do not take clothes off immediately."

《琐碎录》云：若要安乐，不脱不着，北方语也。若要安乐，头脱头着，南方语也。

Suo Sui Lu（《琐碎录》, *Record of Trivials*）says: It is said in northern areas that clothes should not be taken on and off frequently during the seasonal change to stay safe and healthy. It is said in southern areas that clothes should be taken on and off frequently during the seasonal change to stay safe and healthy.

书云：醉酒汗出，脱衣靴袜，当风乘凉，成脚气。

The present book says: Beriberi may be caused if one takes off clothes and shoes and relaxes in a cool place facing the wind when being drunk.

书云：大汗能易衣佳，或急洗亦好。又多汗损血。

The present book says: It is better to change clothes or wash clothes in time when sweating heavily. It also says that excessive sweating damages blood.

又云：大汗偏脱衣，得偏风，半身不遂。又云：劳伤汗出成疾。

It also says: To take off clothes when sweating heavily may lead to

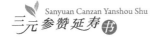
wind stroke and paralysis of half of the body. It also says: Sweating due to overstrain may cause diseases.

书云：大汗急宜敷粉。汗湿衣不可久着，令人发疮及风瘙，大小便不利。

The present book says: Apply powder to the body soon after heavy sweating. Do not wear sweat-soaked clothes for a long time, otherwise it may lead to sores and scabies, abnormal urination and defecation.

书云：汗出毛孔开，勿令人扇，亦为外风所中。又：人汗入诸肉，食之作疔疮。

The present book says: Do not ask others to fan for cool with pores open due to sweating, otherwise it is easy to be invaded by external wind. It also says: Carbuncle may occur if taking meat with sweat in it.

《黄帝素问》曰：饮食饱甚，汗出于胃。饱甚胃满，故汗出于胃也。惊而夺精，汗出于心。惊夺心精，神气浮越，阳内薄之，故汗出于心也；持重远行，汗出于肾。骨劳气越，肾复过疲，故持重远行汗出于肾也。疾走恐惧，汗出于肝。暴役于筋，肝气罢极，故疾走恐惧汗出于肝也。摇体劳苦，汗出于脾。摇动体劳，苦谓动作施力，非疾走远行也，然动作用力则谷精四布，脾化水谷，故汗出于脾也。

Su Wen（《素问》, *Plain Questions*）says: Overeating leads to sweating from the stomach. The reason is that when the stomach is too full, the food qi evaporates and the sweat is generated by the stomach. Fright depletes essence and leads to sweating from the heart. The reason is that when one is frightened, the essence is depleted, the spirit is unsettled, the heart yang is hurt, so sweat is generated by the heart. Going on a long journey with heavy load leads to sweating from the kidney. When traveling with a heavy load, the bone is strained and the qi is excessive, the kidney qi is injured, so sweat is generated by the kidney. Walking in a hurry with fear leads to sweating from the liver. When walking fast in fear, it hurts the sinew, the liver qi is injured and sweat is generated by the liver. Excessive physical work leads to sweating from the spleen. Physical work needs movement and strength which is different with walking fast and far. It depends on the spleen to distribute the food and water, so the spleen qi is injured and sweat is generated by the spleen.

天时避忌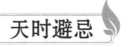

Taboos Related with Climate

《内经》云：阳出则出，阳入则入，无扰筋骨，无见雾露。违此三时，形乃困薄。

Huang Di Nei Jing（《黄帝内经》, *Huangdi's Internal Classic*）says: People's daily routine should keep pace with the time of sunrise and sunset. Do not overwork to avoid damage of the sinew and bones. Do not be exposed to fog and dew. If these three rules were broken, the body physique may become weak and stranded.

《经》云：大寒大热、大风大雾勿冒之。天之邪气，感则害人五脏。水谷寒热，感则害人六腑。地之湿气，感则害人皮肉筋脉。

Jing（《经》, *Classic*）says: Do not get caught in great cold or heat, strong wind or heavy fog. The pathogens from nature can damage the five-zang organs; the cold and heat from food can damage the six-fu organs; the dampness from the earth can damage the skin, muscle, sinews and vessels.

先贤曰：人以一握元气，岂可与大造化敌，康节有四不出之训。

The ancient sages said, "Man cannot go against with nature with his meager original qi." Kang Jie（Shao Kangjie, a philosopher of the Song Dynasty）warned that one ought to stay inside when it is cold, hot, windy and rainy, which is called "Four Kinds of Situations Unsuitable for Going Outside".

书云：犯大寒，而寒至骨髓，主脑逆、头痛、齿亦痛。

The present book says: Extreme cold may invade the marrow and cause the counter-flow of pathogenic factor invading the brain, headache and toothache.

又云：不远热而热至，则头痛、身热、肉痛生矣。

It also says: Failure to keep a distance from heat may bring heat invasion, which can cause headache, fever and pain in the muscle.

真人曰：在家在外，忽逢大风、暴雨、震雷、昏雾，皆是诸龙鬼神经过，宜入室，烧香静坐以避之，过后方出，吉，不尔杀人。

Zhen Ren（Sun Simiao）said, "Strong wind, rainstorm, thunder in the morning or fog in the evening occurring suddenly are thought to be indications that the dragons or ghosts passing by. Whether at home or outside, it is better to enter a room, burn incense, sit quietly, wait until the weather turns fine and then go out. Otherwise, it may lead to disaster."

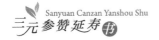

书云：大忌，朔不可哭，晦不可歌，招凶。

The present book says: A great taboo is that one should not cry on the first day of the month or sing on the last day of the month according to the lunar calendar, which can cause inauspicious things.

四时调摄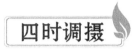

Health Preservation in the Four Seasons

《内经》曰：春三月，此谓发陈，夜卧早起，生而勿杀，逆之则伤肝，夏为寒变，奉长者少。又春伤于风，夏必飧泄。

Huang Di Nei Jing（《黄帝内经》, *Huangdi's Internal Classic*）: The three months of spring is the season of weeding through the old and bringing forth the new and the germination of life. During this period, people should sleep early at night and get up early in the morning. Don't kill indiscriminately. If violating the rule, it can damage the liver and cause cold disease in summer due to insufficient supply for growth. It also says: One will inevitably suffer from lienteric diarrhea in summer if get damaged by wind in spring.

书云：春夏之交，阴雨卑湿，或引饮过多，令犯风湿，自汗体重，转侧难，小便不利。作他治必不救，惟五苓散最佳。

The present book says: At the turn of spring and summer, rheumatism may occur due to rainy whether, dampness of the low-lying land or excessive

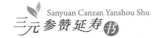
drinking, which may lead to spontaneous sweating, heaviness of the body, inflexibility to turn the body around and difficult urination. In this case, Wuling San（五苓散, Powder of Five Ingredients with Poria）is the best choice to treat the disease and other methods are useless.

《内经》曰：夏三月，此谓蕃秀，夜卧早起，使志无怒，使气得泄。逆之则伤心，秋为疟，奉收者少。

Huang Di Nei Jing（《黄帝内经》, *Huangdi's Internal Classic*）says: The three months of summer is the period of prosperity. People should sleep late at night and get up early in the morning, avoiding any anxiety in life and enabling qi to flow smoothly. Violation of this rule may impair the heart and result in malaria in autumn due to insufficient supply for astringency.

陶隐居云：四时惟夏难将息，伏阴在内腹冷滑。补肾汤剂不可无，食物稍冷休哺啜。

Tao Yinju said, "Among the four seasons, summer is the most difficult one to preserve health. The reason is that internal yin tends to cause abdominal cold and diarrhea. Thus one should take decoctions to tonify the kidney and stay away from cold food."

书云：夏之一季，是人休息之时，心旺肾衰化为水。至秋而凝，冬始坚。当不问老少，皆食暖物，则不患霍乱，腹暖百病不作。

The present book says: Summer is a season for people to have a good rest. At this time, the heart qi is vigorous and the kidney qi is deficient, which can cause the abundance of water inside the body and it becomes condensed in autumn and hardened in winter. Therefore, people of all ages should take warm foods to avoid cholera and keep the abdomen warm to prevent diseases in summer.

书云：夏冰止可隐映饮食，不可打碎食之，入腹冷热相搏成疾。

The present book says: In summer, ice can only be put around to cool down the food instead of being taken directly after being broken into small pieces. Otherwise disease may occur due to the encounter of the cold ice and the warm abdomen.

书云：夏至以后迄秋分，须慎肥腻，饼臛、油酥之属，此物与酒浆、瓜果极理相妨，所以多病者，为此也。

The present book says: From the summer solstice to the autumnal equinox, one should be careful not to eat greasy things such as meat pies or pastries. The reason is that these foods are incompatible with wine syrup and fruits in property, which can cause diseases easily.

陶隐居云：冷枕凉席心勿喜。凡枕冷物大伤人目。

Tao Yinju says, "Do not think it a joy to use cold pillow or bed mat in hot summer." Sleeping with cold pillow damages the eyesight greatly.

书云：夏不宜露卧，令皮肤厚，成癣或作面风。

The present book says: It is not suggested to sleep outside in summer,

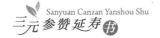

which may cause thick skin, tinea or facial seborrheic dermatitis.

书云：夏伤暑，秋痎疟。忽大寒，勿受之。患时病由此。

The present book says: The heatstroke in summer may lead to malaria in autumn. Keep away from great cold in summer because it might lead to seasonal disease.

书云：暑月日晒处，有石不可便坐，热生疮，冷成疝。

The present book says: It is harmful to sit on the rock burned by sunlight in summer, for the heat of the stone may cause sores and the cold of the stone may lead to hernia.

书云：盛热带汗，当风不宜过。自日中来，勿用冷水沃面，成目疾。伏热者，未得饮水及以冷物迫之，杀人。

The present book says: Do not walk facing wind when in heavy sweat in summer. Do not wash the face with cold water after exposure to the sunlight, which may lead to eye diseases. Those who suffer from latent heat may have the danger of death if not provided with drinking water and cold things to cool down in time.

书云：五六月泽中停水，多有鱼鳖精，饮之成瘕。

The present book says: Most of the ponds are full of water in May and June with semen of fish and turtles. Taking such kind of water might cause abdominal mass.

《内经》曰：秋三月，此谓容平，早卧早起，使志安宁，逆之则伤肺。冬为飧泄，奉藏者少。

Huang Di Nei Jing（《黄帝内经》, *Huangdi's Internal Classic*）says: The three months of autumn is a season of harvest. People should go to bed early and get up early to keep the mind in peace. Any violation of this rule will impair the lung and lead to diarrhea with undigested food in it in winter due to insufficient supply for storage.

书云：秋伤于湿，上逆而咳，发为痿厥。又立秋日勿浴，令皮肤粗燥，因生白屑。又八月一日后，微火暖足，勿令下冷。

The present book says: Damage of dampness in autumn may lead to cough due to reverse flow of qi and atrophy-flaccidity diseases. It also says: Don't take a bath on the beginning day of autumn, otherwise the skin will turn rough and suffer from white crumbs. It also says: After the first day of August according to the lunar calendar, warm the feet with mild fire to keep your lower limbs warm.

《内经》曰：冬三月，此谓闭藏，水冰地拆，无扰乎阳，早卧晚起，必待日光，去寒就温，毋泄皮肤。逆之伤肾，春为痿厥，奉生者少。

Huang Di Nei Jing（《黄帝内经》, *Huangdi's Internal Classic*）says: The three months of winter is the season for storage. The water freezes and the earth cracks. Cares must be taken not to disturb Yang. People should go to bed early and get up late when the sun shines. They should guard themselves

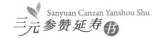
against cold and try to keep warm, avoiding sweating to prevent loss of yang qi. Any violation will impair the kidney and lead to flaccidity and coldness of the limbs in spring due to insufficient supply for growth.

书云：冬时忽大热，勿受之，患时病由此。又曰：冬伤于寒，春必病温。

The present book says: Be cautious of the sudden heat in winter, which may cause seasonal diseases. It also says: Cold damage in winter causes warm diseases in spring.

书云：冬时天地闭，血气藏，作劳不宜，汗出冷背。

The present book says: The whole nature is in the state of storage in winter, so is qi and blood. Therefore, do not overstrain in winter to avoid chilling of back after sweating.

书云：冬寒虽近火，不可令火气聚，不须于火上烘炙，若炙手暖则已，不已损血，令五心热。故手足应于心也。

The present book says: People tend to get warm near the fire in winter, but it is not suggested to centralize fire heat too much and to warm oneself directly above the fire. Stop warming the hands when they are warm enough, otherwise it may cause blood damage and internal heat of the palms, soles and the heart. The reason is that the palms and soles correspond with the heart.

书云：大雪中，跣足人不可便以热汤洗，或饮热酒，足趾随堕。又触寒来，寒未解，勿便饮汤、食热物。

The present book says: After walking barefooted in snow, do not wash the feet with hot water or drink hot wine, otherwise the toes might fall off. It also says: Do not drink hot water or take hot food immediately when the coldness is not released after walking in cold air.

《四气调神论》曰：夫四时阴阳者，万物之根本也。所以圣人春夏养阳，秋冬养阴，与万物浮游于生长之门。逆其根则伐其本，坏其真矣。故阴阳四时者，万物之终始，死生之本也。逆之则灾害生，从之则苛疾不起，是谓得道。故《天真论》曰：有贤人者，逆从阴阳，分别四时，将从上古，合同于道，亦可使益寿而有极时也。

Si Qi Tiao Shen Lun（《四气调神论》, *The Theory of Spiritual Cultivation Conforming with the Four Seasons*）: The changes of yin and yang in the four seasons are the roots of all the things in nature. So the sages cultivate yang in spring and summer while nourish yin in autumn and winter in order to follow such rules. Violation of these rules means destruction of the primordial base and impairment of the body. Thus the changes of yin and yang in the four seasons are responsible for the growth, decline and death of all the things. Any violation of it will bring about disasters. While abidance by it prevents the occurrence of diseases. This is what to follow the law of nature means. Thus, *Shang Gu Tian Zhen Lun*（《上古天真论》, *Ancient Ideas on How to Preserve Natural Health Energy*）says: Sages take care of their bodies according to the changes of yin and yang and the four seasons, which is in line with the ancient way of maintaining health. This can also extend the lifespan to a full limit.

旦暮避忌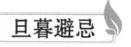

Taboos Concerning Dawn and Dusk

书云：早出含煨生姜少许，辟瘴开胃。又曰：起空腹不宜见尸，臭气入鼻，舌上白起，口臭。欲见，宜饮酒少许。

The present book says: Keeping some simmered ginger in the mouth in the morning can prevent miasma and improve the appetite. It also says: Avoid looking at the corpse with an empty stomach in the morning because the odor of the corpse may lead to white coating of the tongue and stinking smell of the mouth, which can be avoided by drinking some wine before looking at the corpse.

真人曰：平明欲起时，下床先左脚，一日无灾咎，去邪兼辟恶，如能七星步，令人长寿乐。

Zhen Ren（Sun Simiao）said, "When getting up at dawn, the left foot should step on the ground first, which can prevent and ward off various pathogenic factors the whole day. Practice walking in accordance with the Seven-Star Steps in the morning and one can enjoy a long lifespan."

又：清旦常言善事。闻恶事则向所来方三唾之，吉。又：旦勿嗔恚，暮无大醉，勿远行。

He also said, "It is better to talk about auspicious things in the early morning and it brings good luck to spit three times toward the direction from which the bad things are heard. He also said, "Do not get angry and vexed in the morning and do not get drunk or go for a long journey in the evening."

《经》曰：平旦人气生，日中阳气隆，日西阳气已虚，气门乃闭。是故暮而收拒，无扰筋骨，无见雾露。违此三时，形乃困薄。

Huang Di Nei Jing（《黄帝内经》, *Huangdi's Internal Classic*）says: Yang qi becomes active in the morning, flourishes in the noon and declines in the evening and the sweat pores close up accordingly. Thus do not overwork or disturb the sinews and bones or be exposed to fog or dew at dusk. Violation of the movement of yang qi at these three stages（i.e. morning, noon and afternoon）will eventually weaken the body.

书云：夜行用手掠发，则精不敢近。常啄齿，杀鬼邪。又夜卧，二足伸屈不并，无梦泄。

The present book says: When walking outside at night, comb the hair with hands and the pathogens dare not to approach. Knock the teeth often to dispel ghosts and pathogenic factors. It also says: When lying in bed at night, keep one leg stretched and the other bent to prevent nocturnal emission.

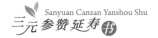

真人云：夜梦恶不须说，且以水面东噀之，咒曰：恶梦着草木，好梦成珠玉。吉。

Zhen Ren（Sun Simiao）said, "Do not talk to others about the nightmares, just spray with water in the mouth toward east and say the cursing words 'The nightmares go to the plants and the good dreams bring jewels.' This can bring good luck."

有教入广者曰：朝不可虚，暮不可实。今气候不齐，不独入广也。

There is a saying for those who have good appetite: Do not have a light diet in the morning and do not eat too much in the evening. Nowadays the climate has changed and the above rule is not only applicable to people with great appetite.

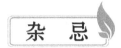

杂 忌

Miscellaneous Taboos

书云：过神庙勿轻入，入必恭谨，不宜恣视，吉。

The present book says: Do not enter the divine temple casually and once inside, remain respectful and cautious, and do not look around arbitrarily, which can bring good luck.

书云：忽见光怪变异之物，强抑勿怪，吉。伊川官廨多妖。有报曰鬼使扇，曰：他热。又曰鬼打鼓，曰：以槌与之。范文正公常读书于府学，每夜有大面之鬼怪近案边。范公以笔书其面曰：汝面非常大，难欺范仲淹。二公不以怪处之，而怪自灭。可为法也。

The present book says: Whenever meeting something strange and bizarre, keep calm and restrained instead of being puzzled and frightened, which can bring good luck. Once ghosts were often seen in the government office of Yichuan, Henan Province. The man on duty reported that the ghost was using the fan. The official replied that he was hot. It was reported again that a ghost was playing the drum. The official replied that hand him the drumstick. Fan Wenzheng used to read at the government school and a ghost with huge face often came near his desk at night. Fan picked up his pen and wrote on his face: Your face is very

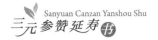
big, but I won't be afraid of you. The two local officials were not scared by the ghosts and they just disappeared by themselves. Their methods can be followed by future generations.

书云：脂油燃灯，人神不安在血光之下。等闲刀画地，乃招不祥事。

The present book says: Lighting a lamp with grease is easy to haunt people and lead to bloodshed. Scribbling on the ground with a knife at will may bring ominous things.

《感应篇》曰：勿朔旦号怒，勿对北恶骂。不可晦腊歌舞，不可对灶吟咏，不可向灶骂詈，不祥。慎勿上床卧歌凶。凡欲眠，勿歌咏，不祥。

Gan Ying Pian（《感应篇》, *The Tract of the Most Exalted on Action and Response*）says: On the first day of each month and in the early morning of each day, do not shout angrily; do not abuse evilly facing the north; do not sing or dance on the last day of each month and Lari（namely, the first day of the first month, the fifth day of May, the seventh day of July, the first day of October and the eighth day of December）; do not chant or curse facing the stove; do not sing when lying in bed, which will bring bad luck; do not sing and chant before falling asleep, which is ominous.

书云：凡刀刃所伤，切勿饮水，令血不止而死。若血不止，急以布蘸热汤盦之，或冷水浸之，嚼寄生叶止血，妙。

The present book says: Whenever one has incised wound, do not drink water, which may lead to death due to endless bleeding. To cure the bleeding, cover it immediately with a cloth soaked with hot water, or put cold water on the wound. It is also effective to stop the bleeding with chewed mistletoe leaves at the same time.

书云：凡古井及深井中多毒气，不可辄入，五六月最甚。先下鸡鸭毛试之，若旋转不下，是有毒气，便不可下去。

The present book says: There might be poisonous gas in the ancient or deep wells, so do not enter them rashly, especially in May and June. Test it by throwing chicken or duck feathers to the wellhead. If the feathers rotate and cannot fall down, there must be poisonous gas in the well and it is forbidden to enter.

又云：山有孔穴。采宝者，惟三月、九月，余月山闭气交死也。

It also says: It is better to go to the mountain with caves to explore and collect treasures in March and September. For the other months, the caves are unventilated with stagnant air, which may cause death due to suffocation.

《琐碎录》云：箫管挂壁取之，勿便吹，恐有蜈蚣。师祖刘复真，赴召早起，见店妇仆地，叫号可畏，但见吹火筒在傍。刘知其蜈蚣入腹，刺猪血灌之，吐出蜈蚣。可不慎欤。

Suo Sui Lu（《琐碎录》, *Record of Trivials*）says: Don't take down the bamboo flute hanging on the wall and blow it promptly in case there may be a centipede in it. The master Liu Fuzhen once got up early in summon to see the Emperor. He saw a female hotel servant lying on the ground and crying terrifyingly. Near the woman there was a blow tube to help ignite fire for cooking. Liu got to know that a centipede hidden in the blow tube was swallowed by the woman. He needled the pig to get its blood and the woman spit out a centipede after drinking the pig blood. How could people be careless about this point!

明·钱塘胡文焕（德父）校
Collated by Hu Wenhuan from Qiantang County of Ming Dynasty

人元之寿 饮食有度者得之

Prolonging Life by Cultivating Ren Yuan

Those Who Keep A Proper Diet Can Achieve It

《黄帝内经》曰："阴之所生，本在五味；阴之五宫，伤在五味。"扁鹊曰："安身之本，必资于食，不知食宜者，不足以存生。"《乡党》一篇具载圣人饮食之节为甚详。后人奔走于名利而饥饱失宜，沉酗于富贵而肥甘之是务，不顺四时，不和五味，而疾生焉。戒乎此，则人元之寿可得矣。

Huang Di Nei Jing（《黄帝内经》, *Huangdi's Internal Classic*）says: Yin is transformed from the five-flavors. The five zang-organs that store yin can also be damaged by the five-flavors. Bian Que said, "Food is the foundation to ensure survival. Health preservation can only be realized by proper diet." *Xiang Dang*（《乡党》, *The Analects of Confucius Hsiang-tang*）recorded in detail the abstinence and taboos of Confucius' diet.

However, people of later generations were busy running about for fame and wealth regardless of their hunger and satiety and engaging themselves in seeking wealth and rank and taking greasy and strong-smelled food without conforming to the changes of the four seasons and harmonizing the five flavors. In this case, diseases may occur. The longevity of human being can be achieved if this lifestyle can be avoided.

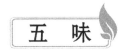

五 味

The Five Flavors

《内经》曰：谨和五味，骨正筋柔，气血以流，腠理以密，长有天命。

Huang Di Nei Jing（《黄帝内经》, *Huangdi's Internal Classic*）says: So only when the five flavors are well balanced can the bones be straightened, the sinews be softened, qi and blood flow smoothly, muscular interstices be intensified and a full natural lifespan be enjoyed.

《淮南子》曰：五味乱口，使口爽，伤病也。

Huan Nan Zi（《淮南子》, *The Huai Nan Zi: A Guide to the Theory and Practice of Government in Early Han China*）says: The five flavors, though complex and delicious, can worsen diseases.

陶隐居云：五味偏多不益人，恐随脏腑成殃咎。五味稍薄，令人神爽，若稍偏多，损伤脏腑，此五行自然之理。初则不觉，久当为患也。

Tao Hongjing（also known as Tao Yinju）said, "Excessive taking of the five flavors is harmful to the health and may damage the corresponding organs. "Moderate-taking of the five flavors is refreshing while excessive taking of them damages the zang-fu organs, which is the natural rule of the five elements. Its impact is not obvious in the early stage but hazardous in the long run.

酸多伤脾，肉胝而唇竭。故春七十二日省酸增甘，以养脾气。

Excessive taking of sour food damages the spleen, wrinkles the skin and turns up the lip. Therefore, people should take less sour food and more sweet food in spring to nourish the spleen qi.

曲直作酸，属木，脾主肉，属土，木克土也。

The liver belongs to wood in the five elements, which has the property of growing freely and pertains to sour in taste. The spleen governs the muscle and belongs to the earth in the five elements. The earth is restricted by the wood.

酸过食，损胃气及肌脏筋骨，不益男子，损颜色。不与蛤同食，相背也。有云：饮少热醋，辟寒胜酒。

Excessive taking of sour food damages the stomach qi, muscle, internal organs, sinews and bones. It is especially harmful to men by worsening the complexion. Sour food is incompatible with clams and they cannot be eaten together. It is also said: Drinking a little vinegar hot can drive away the cold, which is better than wine.

黄戬云：自幼不食醋，今逾八十，尤能传神。

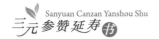
Huang Jian said, "I have never taken vinegar since childhood. Now I am in my eighties and still full of energy."

又：心色赤，宜食酸，小豆、犬肉、李、韭皆酸。

It is also said: The heart corresponds to red in color and favors sour taste. Red beans, dog meat, plums and leeks are sour in taste.

咸多伤心，血凝泣而变色。故冬七十二日，省咸增苦，以养心气。润下作咸，属水，心主血，属火，水克火也。

Excessive taking of salty food damages the heart, which curdles the blood and changes its color. Therefore, people should eat less salty food and more bitter food in winter to nourish the heart qi. The flavor of salt has the function of moistening and flowing downward, which pertains to water in the five elements. The heart governs the blood and pertains to fire in the five elements, which is restrained by water.

盐过于咸，则伤肺，肤黑损筋力。西北人食而耐咸，多寿；东南人食绝欲咸，少寿。病咳及水气者，全宜禁之。

Excessive taking of salt damages the lung, which leads to dark complexion and impaired sinews and muscles. People who take less salt in the Northwest usually enjoy a long lifespan; while people who take much salt in the Southeast tend to have a short lifespan. Those who suffer from cough or edema should keep from taking salt.

晋桃源避世之人，盐味不通，多寿。后五味通而寿啬矣。

People who lived an isolated life in Taoyuan in the Jin Dynasty were long-lived since they had no access to salt. Later, the five tastes of sour, bitter, sweet, spicy and salty were introduced here and people's life expectancy was shorter than before.

又：脾色黄，宜食咸，大豆、豕肉、栗、藿皆咸。

It is also said: The spleen pertains to yellow in color and favors salty food. Soybeans, pork, chestnuts and patchouli are salty in flavor.

甘多伤肾，骨痛齿落，故季月各十八日，省甘增咸，以养肾气。稼穑作甘，属土，肾主骨，属水，土克水也。

Excessive taking of sweet food damages the kidney and leads to pain in bones and shedding of teeth. Thus during the eighteen days in the last month of each season, it is necessary to take less sweet food but more salty food to nourish the kidney qi. The flavor of sweet functions to cultivate and reap and pertains to earth in the five elements. The kidney governs the bones and belongs to water in the five elements, which is restrained by earth.

蜜饧、砂糖，各见本条。

The syrup and sugar belong to this category.

又：肝色青，宜食甘，粳米、牛肉、枣、葵皆甘。

It is also said: The liver pertains to green in color and favors sweet food. Polished round-grained rice, beef, dates and curled mallow are sweet in flavor.

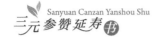
苦多伤肺，皮槁而毛落，故夏七十二曰，省甘增辛，以养肺气。炎上作苦，属火，肺主皮毛，属金，火克金也。

Excessive taking of bitter food damages the lung, which leads to dried skin and loss of hair. Thus people should take less sweet food but more bitter food in summer to nourish the lung qi. The flavor of bitter has the function of flaming up and pertains to fire in the five elements. The lung governs the skin and hair and belongs to the metal in the five elements, which is restricted by fire.

胆、柏皮等。

The gall bladder and arborvitae root bark belong to this category.

又：肺色白，宜食苦，麦、羊肉、杏、薤皆苦。

It is also said: The lung pertains to white in color and favors bitter food. Wheat, mutton, apricot and the Chinese onion are bitter in flavor.

辛多伤肝，筋急而爪枯，故秋七十二曰，省辛增酸，以养肝气。从革作辛，属金，肝主筋，属木，金克木也。

Excessive taking of spicy food damages the liver, which leads to spasm of sinews and dried nails. Thus it is necessary to take less spicy food but more sour food to nourish the liver qi in autumn. The spicy flavor has the function of changing and pertains to metal in the five elements. The liver governs the sinews and pertains to wood in the five elements, which is restrained by metal.

胡椒和气，过多损肺，令人吐血。

Pepper has the function of descending qi, while excessive taking of it damages the lung and leads to blood-spitting.

红椒久食，失明乏气，合口者害人，十月勿食椒，损人心，伤血脉，多忘。除湿温中，益妇人。

Long-time taking of the red pepper leads to blindness and qi deficiency. The one with no cracks is deadly toxic. Do not take pepper in October, which may damage the heart and vessels and lead to poor memory. It has the function of dispelling the dampness and warming the middle, and is beneficial to women.

又：肾色黑，宜食辛，黄黍、鸡肉、桃、葱皆辛。

It also says: The kidney pertains to black in color and favors spicy food. Yellow millet, chicken, peach and scallion are spicy in flavor.

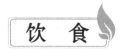

饮 食

Diet

书云：善养性者，先渴而饮，饮不过多，多则损气，渴则伤血。先饥而食，食不过饱，饱则伤神，饥则伤胃。

The present book says: People who are good at health preservation drink water before feeling thirsty. Drinking too much water will damage qi, while being thirsty will damage blood. They eat before feeling hungry and eat to a moderate full. Excessive taking of food will hurt the spirit, while being hungry will damage the stomach.

书云：饮食务取益人者，仍节俭为佳，若过多，觉膨脝短气便成疾。

The present book says: The diet selected should be beneficial to health and be provident. Excessive taking of food may lead to abdominal distention, shortness of breath and disease eventually.

书云：饮食于露天，飞丝堕其中，食之，咽喉生泡。

The present book says: When dining outside, taking food with filament in it may cause blisters in the throat.

书云：饮食收器中，宜下小而上大。若覆之不密，虫鼠欲盗食而不可，环器堕涎。食者得黄病，通身如蜡，针药不能疗。

The present book says: Containers for storing food should be small at the bottom and large at the top to ensure complete covering. If the cover is not tight, insects and mice might drop saliva into food when turning around to steal food. Taking such food may lead to jaundice and the whole body turns yellow as wax, which can not be treated by acupuncture or medicine.

书云：饮食以铜器盖之。汗若入内，食者发恶疮肉疽。

The present book says: Food should be covered with copper utensils. If taking food with sweat dropped into, it may cause severe sores and refractory ulcer.

书云：饮食上蜂行住或猫犬咬破之水，生疮。

The present book says: Drinking water which is touched or licked by bees, cats or dogs may cause sores.

书云：饮食生冷，北人土厚水深，禀气坚实，不损脾胃。久居南方，宜忌之。南人土薄水浅，禀赋多虚，不宜脾胃。久居北方者，尤宜忌之。

The present book says: People living in northern areas have strong constitution due to the fertile soil and deep water, so the taking of raw and cold food will not damage their spleen and stomach. But they should be

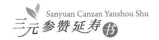

cautious not to take raw and cold food if living in southern areas for a long time. People living in southern areas have weak constitution due to barren soil and shallow water, so the taking of raw and cold food will damage the spleen and stomach. They should be cautious not to take raw and cold food if living in northern areas for a long time.

书云：空心茶，宜戒；卯时酒、申后饭，宜少。

The present book says: It should be forbidden to drink tea on an empty stomach and be restrained to drink wine at Mao Shi（the period of the day from 5 a.m. to 7 a.m.）and eat after Shen Shi（the period of the day from 3 p.m. to 5 p.m.）.

书云：极饥而食且过饱，结积聚极。渴而饮且过多，成痰癖。日没后食讫，便未须饮酒，不干呕。

The present book says: When being excessively hungry, eating to the degree of satiety may lead to accumulation and stagnation in the body. When being excessively thirsty, drinking too much water may lead to phlegm. Dinner should be finished after sunset and one will not retch if keeping away from drinking wine at this time.

太宗谓宰臣曰："朕每日所为，自有常节，饮食不过度，行之已久，甚觉有力。老子云：'我命在我，不在天，全在人之调适。'卿等亦当加意，毋自轻摄养也。"

The Emperor Taizong of the Song Dynasty told his Prime Minister, "My daily routine is very regular and I never take food excessively, which has been kept on for a long time and makes me energetic. Lao Zi once said that his fate was determined by himself instead of the Heaven and one's lifespan depended on one's own regulation. You should also be devoted to preserve health and do not neglect its effect."

陶隐居云：何必餐霞服大药，妄意延年等龟鹤。但于饮食嗜欲中，去其甚者将安乐。

Tao Yinju said, "Don't have to take the so-called elixirs to extend the lifespan as long as turtle and crane. Just keep a moderate diet and a peaceful and indifferent mind to desires, the goal of happiness and longevity can be realized."

浆水，按《本草》，味甘酸，微温，无毒。调中引气，开胃止渴，强力通关，治霍乱泻痢。消宿食，解烦去睡，调理脏腑，治呕哕，白人肤体如缯帛。为人常用，故不齿其功。

Jiang Shui（starch solution, processed with corn and fermented）, according to *Ben Cao*（《本草》, *Classic of Materia Medica*）, is sweet and sour in taste, and slightly warm in property, nontoxic. It has the function of regulating the middle and guiding qi downward, stimulating the appetite and relieving thirst, and dredging the obstruction. It is used to treat cholera, dysentery, indigestion, vexation and somnolence, regulate zang-fu organs, relieve vomiting and hiccup, and whiten the skin as smooth as the silk. Since it is commonly used in daily life, its efficacy is underestimated.

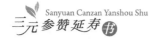

世之所用熟水品目甚多，贵如沉香则燥脾，木骨草则涩气，蜜香则冷胃，麦门冬则体寒，如此之类，皆有所损。

There are many kinds of boiled water used in daily life. That made by expensive medicinal materials, such as Chenxiang [沉香, Aquilaria, Aquilariae Lignum Resinatum] can dry the spleen, that made by Mugucao [木骨草, Common Scouring Rush Herb, Herba Equiseti Hiemalis] can astringe qi, that made by honey aroma can cause cold in the stomach, and that made by Maimendong [麦门冬, Radix Ophiopogonis, Ophiopogon Japonicus Ker-Gawl] can lead to body cold. Such kinds of boiled water are harmful to the body.

紫苏汤，今人朝暮饮之，无益也。芳草致豪贵之疾，此有一焉。宋仁宗命翰林院定熟水，奏曰："紫苏第一，沉香第二，麦门冬第三。以苏能下胸膈浮气。"殊不知久则泄人真气，令人不觉。

The decoction of purple perilla is taken by people in the morning and evening presently, which is harmful actually. Improper taking of medicinal herbs may cause diseases among the rich and noble, and purple perilla is a case in point. The Emperor Renzong of the Song Dynasty ordered the Imperial Academy to decide the boiled water for him to drink. They reported, "Purple perilla ranks the first, agilawood the second, and radix ophiopogonis the third. The reason is that purple perilla can descend the floating qi in the chest and diaphragm." It is hardly realized that long-time drinking of this water will discharge the genuine qi unconsciously.

《本草》云：酒饮之，体软神昏，是其有毒也，损益兼行。

Ben Cao (《本草》, *Classic of Materia Medica*) says: Excessive drinking of wine leads to physical weakness and loss of consciousness, which indicates that it is toxic. Moderate drinking of it is beneficial while excessive drinking is harmful to the health.

扁鹊云：久饮常过，腐肠烂胃，溃髓蒸筋，伤神损寿。

Bian Que said, "Long-term and excessive drinking of wine leads to corroded stomach and intestine, ulcerated marrow, steamed sinews, exhausted spirit and shortened lifespan."

有客访周顗，顗出美酒两石，顗饮石二，客饮八斗。次明，顗无所苦，酒量贯也，客已死矣。观之，客肠已出，胁已穿。岂非量过，而犯扁鹊之戒欤？

Once a guest visited Zhou Yi and Zhou Yi took out two Dan of good-quality wine, of which Zhou Yi drank one Dan and two Dou, the guest drank eight Dou. The next morning, Zhou Yi was fine since he always drank like this while his guest was already dead. When examining, it was found out that the intestines of the guest were out, and his ribs were penetrated. Is it not because of the excessive taking of wine that violates Bian Que's warning?

饮白酒，食牛肉，生虫。酒浆照人无影，不可饮。不可合乳汁饮，令人气结。祭酒自耗者杀人。酒后食芥辣物，多则缓人筋骨。

To drink liquor and take beef at the same time may cause parasites in the stomach. Do not drink the wine if the image of people can't be reflected in it. Do not drink liquor mixed with milk at the same time, which will lead to qi stagnation. To drink the liquor used for sacrifice may lead to death. To take excessive spicy food such as mustard after drinking makes the sinews

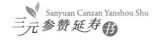
and bones lassitude.

卧黍穰，食猪肉，患大风。凡中药毒及一切毒，从酒得者难治。酒性行血脉，流遍身体也。

To take pork on the millet stalk may cause severe stroke. It is hard to treat medicinal and other kinds of toxicity induced by wine. The reason is that wine enters the vessel and circulates around the whole body.

书云：饮酒醉未醒，大渴饮冷水，又饮茶，被酒引入肾脏，为停毒之水。腰脚重腿，膀胱冷痛，兼患水肿，消渴挛痹。

The present book says: To relieve thirsty by drinking cold water and tea with a hangover may cause stagnation of toxic water in the kidney conducted downward by wine. This may lead to symptoms like heaviness and swelling of waist and feet, cold and pain of the bladder, edema, diabetes and spastic paralysis.

书云：酒醉当风，以扇扇之，恶风成紫瘢。又：醉酒吐罢，便饮水，作消渴。神仙不禁酒，以能行气壮神，然不过饮也。

The present book says: To face the wind or fan for cool after getting drunk, one may suffer from purpura. It also says: Drink water immediately after vomiting due to drunk may cause diabetes. Immortals also drink occasionally to promote qi circulation and strengthen the spirit, but they never drink excessively.

《本草》：茶饮者，宜热，宜少，不饮尤佳。久食去人脂，令人瘦，下焦虚冷。唯饱食后一二盏不妨消渴也。饥则尤不宜，令人不眠。同韭食身重。

Ben Cao（《本草》, *Classic of Materia Medica*）says: It is better to drink hot tea in proper amount and it is best to drink none of it. Long-time drinking of tea can remove fat, keep slim, cause deficiency and cold in the lower energizer. It can relieve thirsty to drink one or two cups of tea after dinner. It is especially inappropriate to drink tea in the state of hunger, which can lead to insomnia. To take leeks while drinking tea makes the body heavy.

书云：将盐点茶，引贼入家，恐伤肾也。

The present book says: Putting salt into tea is like inviting a thief home since it's harmful to the kidney.

东坡《茶说》：除烦去腻，世固不可无茶。然暗中损人不少，吾有一法常自修之。辄以浓茶漱口于食后，烦腻既去而脾胃不知。凡肉之在齿者，得茶漱涤，乃不觉脱去，不烦挑剔也。盖齿性便苦，缘此渐坚牢，而齿蠹且日去矣。

Cha Shuo（《茶说》, *On Tea*）by Su Dongpo says: Tea drinking is indispensable for removing greasiness. However, drinking tea is also harmful to health unconsciously. I have a method to make good use of tea in practice. That is to gargle with tea after dinner to relieve greasiness and protect the spleen and stomach meanwhile. Meat scraps stuffed between the teeth can also be rinsed with tea easily without troubling to scrape off. Probably

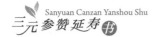
the property of teeth is compatible with the bitter flavor, so the practice of gargling mouth with tea can gradually strengthen the teeth and remove the tooth decay.

书云：饮多，则肺布叶举，气逆上奔。

The present book says: Excessive drinking of tea can cause the lung lobes lifted up and the counter flow of qi.

书云：阴地流泉，六月行路，勿饮之，发疟。

The present book says: Do not drink water of the stream-let in the graveyard in June, which can cause malaria.

书云：饮宴于圣像之侧，魂魄不安。

The present book says: Enjoying a feast beside the statue of a sage can get the soul and spirit disturbed.

书云：饮水勿急咽，久成气病。

The present book says: Do not drink water hastily, which may lead to qi disorder in the long run.

书云：形寒饮冷，则伤肺，上气咳嗽，鼻鸣。

The present book says: Drinking cold water when the body is freezing damages the lung and leads to cough and snorting nose due to the counter-flow of qi.

书云：粥后饮白汤，为淋，为停湿。

The present book says: Drinking boiled water after porridge can cause strangury and retention of dampness.

陶隐居云：食戒欲粗并欲速，宁可少餐相接续。莫教一饱顿充肠，损气伤心非尔福。

Tao Yinju said, "It is better to eat moderately and frequently rather than swallow roughly and hastily. Keep away from excessive full stomach, which may damage qi and the heart and bring trouble."

《养生》云：美食须热嚼，生肉不须吞。

Yang Sheng（《养生》, *Health Preservation*）says: Delicious food should be taken warm and chewed finely, and meat should not be swallowed raw.

又云：食毕漱口数过，齿不龋，口不臭。漱口忌热汤，则损牙齿。

It also says: Rinse the mouth several times after dinner and then the teeth will not be decayed and the mouth will not be stinking. Do not rinse with hot water, which may damage the teeth

又云：食炙煿宜待冷，不然伤血脉，损齿。

It also says: Wait till the roasted meat cool down before eating, otherwise it may damage the blood, the vessel and the teeth.

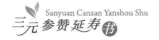

书云：食厨屋漏水堕脯肉，成癥瘕，生恶疮。

The present book says: If taking the dried meat with rain water leaked from the roof, abdominal mass and sores may occur.

书云：人汗入肉，食之作疗疮。又，食诸兽自死肉亦然。

The present book says: If taking meat with sweat dropped on, furuncle and sores may occur. It also says: It is also true if taking meat of naturally dead animals.

书云：食物以象牙、金铜为匙箸，可以试毒。

The present book says: Toxicity of food can be tested by using spoons or chopsticks made of ivory, gold or copper.

隐居云：生冷黏腻筋韧物，自死牲牢皆勿食。馒头闭气莫过多，生脍偏招脾胃疾。炸酱胎卵兼油腻，陈臭淹藏尽阴类。老人朝暮更餐之，借是寇兵无以异。

Tao Yinju said, "Don't take raw, cold, sticky, greasy, and tough food, or naturally dead livestock. Don't take too much steamed bread, otherwise it may cause stagnation of qi. Don't take raw meat, otherwise it may cause disorder of the spleen and stomach. Fried or pickled egg fetuses are greasy, stale and smelly foods stored for a long long pertain to yin. If the elderly people take these foods in the morning and evening, the damage to their health is the same as inviting enemies to their houses."

《琐碎录》云：馒头闭气悔血，汤以破之。包子包气，好醋以破之。

Suo Sui Lu（《琐碎录》, *Record of Trivials*）says: The steamed bread leads to stagnation of qi and blood, which can be avoided by taking soup. The steamed stuffed bun blocks qi in the organs, which can be avoided by taking vinegar.

书云：食物以鱼鲩器盛之，有蛊毒，辄裂破。入闽者，宜审之。

The present book says: Use the vessel made of fish head bones to hold food, which may break if there is poison in the food produced by venomous insects. Those who enter into Fujian should be cautious with this.

书云：夜半之食宜戒，申酉前晚食为宜。

The present book says: Quit the habit of eating at midnight. Dinners should be taken before Shen Shi（three to five o'clock in the afternoon）and You Shi（five to seven o'clock in the afternoon）.

《周礼》：乐以消食。

Zhou Li（《周礼》, *The Chou Rituals*）says: The sound of music is beneficial for digesting food.

盖脾喜音声，夜食则脾不磨，为音响绝也。夏月夜短，尤宜忌之。

The reason is that the spleen favors sound and it does not function well at night when everything is silent. It is especially not suitable to eat at night in summer since the night time is

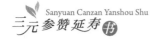

shorter than other seasons.

老子云：不饥强食，则脾劳。不渴强饮，则胃胀。食欲常少，勿令虚。冬则朝勿虚，夏则夜勿饱。

Lao Zi said, "Do not manage to eat if not hungry, otherwise it may lead to over-strain of the spleen. Do not manage to drink if not thirsty, otherwise it may lead to distention of the stomach. Do eat moderately and frequently and keep the stomach from being empty. In winter, keep the stomach from being empty in the morning, while in summer, keep the stomach from being full at night."

书云：君子慎言语，节饮食。人之当食，须去烦恼。食毕当漱口数过，令人牙齿不败，口香。

The present book says: A gentleman should be cautious with his words and moderate in his diet. Forget the annoyance when having dinners. Rinse the mouth several times after meals to protect the teeth from decaying and freshen the breath.

天隐子云：人之有斋戒者，斋乃洁净之物，戒乃节慎之称。有饥即食，食勿全饱，此所谓中也。百味未成熟，勿食，五味太多，勿食，腐败闭气之物，勿食，此皆宜戒也。手常摩擦皮肤，温热熨去冷气，此所谓畅外也。此是调理形骸之法。

Tian Yinzi said, "For those who are on a period of fasting, which refers to keeping clean and abstaining from desires, they eat only when hungry and eat moderately, which is called moderation. Do not take anything uncooked; do not take anything flavored excessively with the five tastes; do not take anything putrid and qi-stagnating. All these should be forbidden. Rub the skin warm with hands often to expel the cold qi, which makes the external circulation unobstructed. This is the method to regulate the body."

书云：色恶不食，臭恶不食，失饪不食，不时不食。前云：色臭二恶不食者，谓饭食及肉颜色香臭变恶者，皆不食之。失饪不食者，谓非朝、夕、日中时也。

The present book says: Don't take food with abnormal color or food with stinking smell or food cooked inappropriately or food at inappropriate time. The former two conditions refer to the color and smell of the food and meat have been bad which is inedible. The latter two conditions refer to taking meals irregularly instead of at the proper time of morning, noon and evening.

书云：饮食以时，饥饱得中，水谷变化，冲气和融，精血生，荣卫以行，腑脏调平，神志安宁，正气充实于内，元真通会于外。内外邪沴莫之能干，一切疾患无从所作也。又：饮食之宜，当候已饥而进食，食不厌熟嚼；仍候焦渴而引饮，饮不厌细呷。无待饥甚而后食，食不可饱；或觉微渴而省饮，饮不欲太频。食不厌精细，饮不厌温热。

The present book says: To have a regular diet and moderate amount of food can ensure the normal transformation of food and smooth circulation of qi, which can generate essence and blood, promote the normal circulation

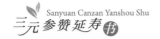

of nutrient and defensive qi, regulate the zang-organs and fu-organs, calm the mind and spirit, strengthen the healthy qi internally and primordial qi externally, resist pathogenic factors from inside or outside and prevent various diseases. It also says: Eat only when hungry and chew slowly and fully; Drink only when thirsty and drink with moderate amount each time. Don't wait to eat when extremely hungry and do not eat too full; Drink when slightly thirsty and do not drink too frequently. Food should be taken as careful as possible and water should be drunk as warm as possible.

食无生冷、坚韧、焦燥、粘滑物伤，则胃中水谷易于腐化矣。食物饱甚，耗气非一，或食不下而上涌呕吐以耗灵源，或饮不消而作痰咯唾以耗神水。

Don't take raw, cold, hard, dry, burnt or sticky food, and then the food is easy to digest in the stomach. It consumes qi if eating too much, exhausts spirit if vomiting due to the up-welling of undigested food, consumes body fluid if spitting phlegm and saliva due to the failure of fluid circulation.

好食炙煿者，将为口疮、咽痛、壅热、痈疡之疾。

Those who like to take fried or roasted food are prone to suffer from aphtha, sore throat, fever due to stagnation or carbuncle and ulcer.

偶食物饱甚，虽觉体倦，无辄就寝，可运动徐行纳百余步，然后解带、松衣、伸腰、端坐，两手按摩心腹，交叉来往约一二十过，复以两手自心胁间按擦，向下约十数过，令心腹气道不至壅塞，过饱食随手消化也。

当盛暑时，食饮加意调节，缘伏阴在内，腐化稍迟。又：果蓏园蔬，多将生啖，苏水桂浆，唯欲冷饮，生冷相值，克化尤难。微伤即飧泄，重伤即霍乱吐利。是以暑月食物尤要节减，使脾胃易于磨化，戒忌生冷，免有腹脏之疾也。

An occasional full stomach may lead to tiredness, and it can be relieved by this method: keep from going to bed early, walk slowly for about 100 steps, take off clothes, stretch the back, sit upright, massage the heart and abdomen with hands for about 10 to 20 times, then rub downward from the heart to the ribs with hands for about 10 times to keep the qi circulation smooth and digest the food overtaken timely. In midsummer, one should pay more attention to the regulation of diet because yin qi is stored inside at this time and the digestion speed of food slows down slightly. It also says: In summer, vegetables and fruits are mostly taken raw. Perilla juice and laurel syrup are usually drunk cold. The raw food and the cold drink are often intertwined, which makes it especially difficult to digest. Thus it may lead to diarrhea if the damage is slight and cholera and vomiting if the damage is severe. Therefore, diet should be carefully regulated in summer to conform to the digesting function of the spleen and stomach. Raw and cold food should be avoided in summer to prevent disorders of the abdomen.

《琐碎录》云：暑月瓷器如日照者，不可便盛饮食。

Suo Sui Lu（《琐碎录》, *Record of Trivials*）says: Porcelain vessels cannot be used to hold food immediately after being exposed to sunshine in summer.

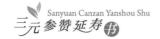
阎孝忠曰：吴楚之人，每中脘有疾，悉谓脾病，胸腹痛不以虚实，悉谓脾病。凡脾药皆椒姜术附之类。又盛夏必热食，居密室服药，习以为常。余劝以夏当寒食高居，以远炎暑。则曰：吴楚与北人异。以此自将，安乐充实，岂不难哉。《经》云：春夏养阳，秋冬养阴，顺天地之柔刚。注：阴报于阳谓五月，五阳一阴始生，圣人春食温，夏食寒，以抑阳扶阴。十一月，五阴一阳，故热附炎，以抑阴扶阳，反此者是谓伐根。盛夏热食，穷冬寒食，以自取困踣，吾末如之何。

Yan Xiaozhong said, "For the local residents of Wu and Chu, they regarded the disorder of the middle part of gastric cavity as rooted from the spleen disorder and the chest or abdominal pain as rooted from the spleen disorder without differentiation of its excess or deficiency. The drugs for treating spleen disorder are nothing more than pepper, Shengjiang [生姜, Fresh Ginger, Rhizoma Zingiberis Recens], Baizhu [白术, Largehead Atractylodes Rhizome, Rhizoma Atractylodis Macrocephalae], Fuzi [附子, Prepared Common Monkshood Daughter Root, Radix AconitiLateralis Preparat] and the like. Moreover, the residents usually take food warm in midsummer and take medicine in a closed room. I once persuaded them to take more cool foods and stay in higher places in summer to relieve the heat. They answered: that they are different from northerners. To preserve health in this way can hardly help to achieve happiness and health. *Huang Di Nei Jing* (《黄帝内经》, *Huangdi's Internal Classic*) says: Yang qi is cultivated in spring and summer and yin qi is cultivated in autumn and winter so as to adapt to the changes of cold and heat in the four seasons. Note: In May, the yin within yang begins to prosper and the sage takes warm food in spring and cold food in summer to restrain yang and support yin. In November, the yang within yin begins to prosper and the sage makes use of heat to raise yang and restrain yin. Those who do the opposite rock the fundamentals of the body. Taking hot food in midsummer and cold food in winter can bring lots of trouble, which I do not have any idea to deal with."

一日之忌暮无饱，食物至饱伤脏腑。又：人之阳气，随日升沉，日中则隆，日西则虚。无劳复筋骨，当休息肢体，力省运行，食难磨化，或即就寝，不免重伤。故云：夜食饱甚，损一日之寿也。

Don't eat too much for supper, which may damage the viscera. It also says: Yang qi in the human body changes with the sunrise and sunset. It is abundant at noon and deficient at sunset. At this time, do not overstrain and relax the body properly to have a good rest. To go to bed with undigested food in the stomach may lead to great damage to the body. Thus as the saying goes: Taking an excessive amount of food at night may lose one day's lifespan.

王叔和洞识摄生之道，常谓：人日食不欲杂，杂则或有所犯，当时或无灾患，积久为人作疾。寻常饮食，每令得所，多食令人膨脝短气，或致暴疾。夏至秋分，少食肥腻、饼臛之属。此物与酒食瓜果相妨，当时不必习病，入秋节变，阳消阴息，寒气总至，多诸暴卒。良由涉夏取冷太过，饮食不节故也。而不达者，皆以病至之日便谓是受病之始，而不知其所由来者渐矣。岂不惑哉？

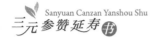
Wang Shuhe had a deep understanding of the way to maintain health. He often said, "The daily diet should not be too miscellaneous, otherwise it may lead to incompatibility among the foods and though there is no immediate danger then, it can result in diseases in the long run. Take proper amount of foods in daily life, otherwise it may cause abdominal distention and shortness of breath, or even acute diseases. From the summer solstice to the autumn equinox, take less greasy food or meat pies because they are similar with drinks and fruits and though safe then, can lead to acute diseases due to the waning of yang and waxing of yin and the arrival of cold qi in autumn. It is because of excessive taking of raw and cold food and improper diet in summer. Those who don't understand the truth behind it think that the onset time of disease is the time for its occurrence without the knowledge about the gradual development of the disease. How can they not be confused!"

.

食 物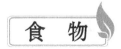

Food

物之无益而有损者，常人尤不可多食，况病人当避忌者乎？此书所载，凡物之有益而无损者，不书。或损益相半者，则书其损而不书其益。

Those foods that are harmful to health should not be taken by ordinary people, let alone patients. Those foods that are beneficial for health are not recorded in this book. For those foods that are both beneficial and harmful to health, their harmful aspects are recorded in this book only.

果 实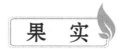

Fruits

生枣令人热渴气胀，寒热。羸瘦者，弥不可多。动脏腑，损脾元。与蜜同食损五脏。

Taking raw dates can cause thirst due to heat, qi distention and chills and fever. Those who are weak should not take them excessively, otherwise it may disturb the viscera and damage the essence of the spleen. Taking it together with honey impairs the five zang-organs.

软枣冷，动宿疾，发嗽，与蟹相忌。

Black date is cold in property and is prone to cause abiding disease and cough. It is incompatible with crabs.

梅子坏齿及筋，多食发热。

Plum damages the teeth and sinews and excessive taking of it leads to fever.

生龙眼平，沸汤内淖过不动脾。

Raw longan is mild in property and the blanched ones will not disturb the spleen.

樱桃，寒热病多食，发暗风，伤筋骨，呕吐。小儿多食作热，性热也。

Excessive taking of cherries for patients with cold-heat syndrome can cause dizziness, damage of sinews and bones and vomiting. Excessive taking of it for children may cause fever due to its heat property.

生荔枝性热，多食发虚热、烦渴、口干、衄血。

The raw litchi is heat in property, thus excessive taking of it can lead to deficiency-heat, polydipsia, thirst，dryness in the mouth and nose bleeding.

楂子不可多食，损齿及筋。

Excessive taking of hawthorn can damage the teeth and sinews.

乳柑太寒，冷脾，发痼疾，利肠，发轻汗。脾胃冷人，尤不可多食，诸柑性同。

Ru Gan（Citrus produced in Wenzhou with the taste of cheese）is very cold in property, thus it can lead to cold of the spleen, arouse abiding diseases, dredge the intestines and induce slight sweat. Those with cold in the stomach and spleen should not take an excessive amount of it. All kinds of citrus have the same property.

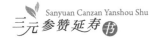

橘柚酸者聚痰，甜者润肺，不可多食，令人口爽，不知五味。

Sour tangelo produces phlegm and sweet one nourishes the lung. Though it can refresh the mouth, it should not be overtaken for it can make people unable to recognize the five kinds of flavors.

橙子温，皮多食伤肝，与槟榔同食，头旋恶心，生痰作疟。

Orange is warm in property and excessive taking of its peel damages the liver. Taking it together with areca-nut can cause dizziness, nausea, produce phlegm and lead to malaria.

杨梅多食发热，损齿及筋。

Excessive taking of waxberry generates heat and damages the teeth and sinews.

杏实热，多食伤筋骨。杏酥生熟吃俱得，半生半熟，杀人。杏仁久服，目盲，眉、发、须落，动宿疾。双仁者，杀人，可研细治犬伤。

Apricot is heat in property and excessive taking of it damages the sinews and bones. Almond cookies can be taken both raw and cooked, but the half-cooked ones are deadly to take. Long-time taking of almonds leads to blindness, loss of eyebrow, hair and beard, and arouses the abiding disease. The ones with double kernels are deadly to take, but they can be applied on dog bites after grinding to powder.

桃实发丹石，损胃，多食有热。饱食桃仁，水浴成淋。

The peach nut generates the toxicity of elixir and damages the stomach. Taking an excessive amount of it produces heat. Bathing after taking the peach kernels too much causes strangury。

桃杏花本五出，而六出者，必双仁，能杀人者，失常故也。

The flowers of peach and apricot usually have five petals, while those with six petals must have double kernels and are deadly to take, since they are abnormal in morphology.

李子，平，发疟，多令虚热，白蜜和食，伤人五内。不可临水上啖之及与雀肉同食。李不沉水者，毒。仁和鸡子食，内结不消。

Plum is mild in property and can cause malaria and deficiency-heat. Taking it together with whitish honey damages the five zang-organs. Do not take it near water or together with sparrow meat. Those that float on water are poisonous. Taking the plum kernels together with eggs causes indigestion and internal stagnation.

梨寒，乳鹅梨、紫花梨治心热，此外生不益人，多食，寒中。产妇、金疮人勿食，令萎困。其性益齿而损脾胃，正、二月勿食佳。

Pear is cold in property. Ru'e pear and Zihua Pear can be used to treat heart heat and the other kinds of it are not suitable for taking raw, which may cause cold damage to the middle part of the body. Puerpera and those with incised wound are forbidden to take pears, which can make them weak and depressed. It brings benefit to the teeth but harm to the spleen and the

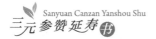
stomach. Do not take it during the first and second month of the year.

藤梨，名沐猴梨，食多冷中。

Chinese gooseberry is also called Muhou pear. Taking an excessive amount of it can damage the middle with its coldness.

林檎多食，发热涩气，好睡发冷疾，生疮疖，脉闭不行，子不可食，令人烦。

Taking an excessive amount of Chinese pear-leaved crabapple can generate heat and astringe qi, cause somnolence and diseases due to cold, sores and furuncles, and blocked vessels. Its seeds can not be taken for it may cause vexation.

石榴多食，损肺及齿。山石榴多无益，涩气。

Taking an excessive amount of pomegranate damages the lung and the teeth. The wild ones usually bring no benefit to health due to their function of astringing qi.

栗子，温，生治腰脚。生即发气，宜暴干蒸炒。食多即气壅，患风水气人不宜食。生栗可于灰火中煨令汗出，杀其水气，不得通熟。小儿食生者，多难化。熟者，多滞气。

Chestnut is warm in property and the raw ones can treat the diseases of the waist and feet. The raw ones can cause gastric distension, thus they should be dried, fried and steamed before eating. Excessive taking of it leads to qi stagnation so they are not suitable for people with wind-edema. The raw chestnuts can be baked in the hot ash till they are dry but not fully cooked. The raw ones are difficult to digest and the cooked ones are qi-stagnating for children.

柿子，寒，日干者，性冷，多食腹痛，生者弥冷。红柿与蟹同食，吐红。饮酒食红柿，心痛至死，亦易醉，不解酒毒。一种塔柿引痰，日干多动风火，干味不佳。

Persimmon is cold in property. Those dried under sunshine are cold in property which may lead to pain in the abdomen if taking excessively. The unripe ones are especially cold in property. Taking the red ones together with crabs leads to hematemesis, and together with wine leads to deadly pain in the heart, susceptibility to drunk and difficulty to relieve wine toxicity. The kind of persimmon shaped like a tower tends to produce phlegm. Those dried under sunshine can cause wind-fire syndrome and those dried ones are not tasty.

椑子性尤冷，与蟹同食，腹疼大泻。

Beizi, a kind of smaller persimmon, is especially cold in property, and taking it together with crab leads to pain in the abdomen and severe diarrhea.

葡萄酒过，昏人眼。架下饮酒，防虫屎伤人。

Grapes macerated in wine can lead to blurred vision. Be cautious of insect droppings while drinking wine under the grape trellis.

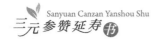

白果生引疳,解酒。熟食益人,然不可多食,腹满。有云:满一千个者,死。此物二更开花,三更结子,当是阴毒之物。

The raw gingko can cause infantile malnutrition and has the function of dispelling the effect of wine. The cooked ones are beneficial to health but the excessive taking of it can cause distension of the abdomen. It is said that taking a thousand of gingkoes may cause death. It blooms at the second watch of the night（9-11 p.m.）and bears fruits at the third watch of the night（11 p.m.-1 a.m.）, so it is the fruit with yin toxin.

有人艰籴,取白果以为饭,饱食,次日皆死。

Those who were lack of food and took gingkoes as food till full, were all found dead the next day.

菱芰也冷脏, 色利损阳, 令阴萎, 不益脾, 难化, 令胀满, 姜酒解之。七月食生菱, 作蛲虫。

Water chestnut can cause cold damage to the viscera, bring diarrhea, damage of yang, impotence, damage to the spleen and distension, which can be relieved by ginger wine. Taking the raw ones at July might cause pinworms.

茨菰, 大寒, 动宿冷气, 腹胀满, 小儿秋食之, 脐下痛, 孕不可食。吴茱萸食, 患脚气, 瘫痪, 损齿, 失颜色。

Arrowhead is greatly cold in property which can arouse the abiding cold in the body and causes distension of the abdomen. Children who take it in autumn suffer from pain under the navel. It is forbidden to eat for the pregnant. Fructus evodiae tend to induce beriberi, paralysis, loss of teeth and poor complexion.

荸荠性与乌芋同。

The property of Chinese water chestnut is the same as black taro.

芡实生食，动风冷气，损脾难消却益精。

Taking the raw gorgon can disturb internal wind and the cold qi, damage the spleen and lead to indigestion. It is beneficial to the essence.

藕多食，冷中，能去疫气。产后惟此不同生冷忌者，破血故也。

Lotus root can be taken to cool the middle and dispel pestilent qi. It is forbidden to take raw and cold food after childbirth, but the lotus root is an exception because of its function of removing blood stasis.

甜瓜动痼疾，多食，阴下湿痒，生疮，发虚热，破腹，令人惙惙弱，脚手无力。少食则可不中暑，多食未有不下。贫下多食，深秋下痢难治，损阳故也。患脚气食此，永不除。五月甜瓜沉水者，杀人。多食，发黄疸，动气，解药力。双蒂者，杀人。与油饼同食发病。

Taking melon can arouse chronic disease, and excessive taking of it leads to genital pruritus due to dampness, sores, deficiency-heat, diarrhea, and fatigue and weakness of limbs. Moderate taking of it can relieve summer-

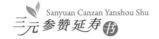
heat, while excessive taking of it leads to diarrhea. The poor people who take an excessive amount of it may suffer from dysentery in autumn which is hard to cure due to yang damage. Those who suffer from beriberi find it hard to cure if taking it. The melons that sink in the water in May are deadly to eat. Excessive taking of it leads to jaundice, qi disturbance and reduces the efficacy of medicinals. Melons with double pedicels are deadly to take. Taking it together with deep-fried dough cake causes diseases.

防州太守陈逢原，避暑食瓜至秋，忽腰腿痛，不能举动，遇商助教疗之，更生。

Chen Fengyuan, who was the prefecture chief of Fangzhou, took melons a lot to get cool in summer till autumn and suffered from pain in the legs and waist, unable to move. The merchant he met taught him how to treat it, and he got recovered.

西瓜甚解暑毒，北人禀厚食惯，南人禀薄，不宜。多食至于霍乱、冷病，终身不除。

Watermelon can relieve the summer-heat. The northerners have strong constitution, so they are accustomed to eating them. While the southerners have weak constitution, so watermelons are not fit for them. Excessive taking of it can lead to cholera or cold damage, which can not be cured the whole life.

木瓜，温，皮薄微赤黄，香，甘酸不涩，向里子头尖，一面方，是真。益脾而损齿。若圆和，子微黄，蒂粗，涩。小圆，味涩微咸，伤人气，多食损牙。

Pawpaw is mild in property with thin and yellowish peel. It is fragrant in smell and sweet and sour in taste. Those with one sharp point inside and the other square are of good quality. It is beneficial to the spleen while harmful to the teeth. If it is round-shaped with slightly yellowish seeds and thick pedicle, it is acerbic in taste. If it is small and round, it is acerbic and salty in taste which damages qi and impairs the teeth if taking excessively.

甘蔗多食，衄血。烧其滓，烟入目则眼暗。

Excessive taking of sugar canes can lead to nose bleeding. When burning the residue of it, the smoke leads to blurred vision.

砂糖，寒，多食心痛。鲫同食成疳；葵同食生流癖；笋同食成食癥，身重不能行。小儿多食，损齿及生蛲虫。

Sugar is cold in property and excessive taking of it leads to heartache. Taking it together with carp leads to infantile malnutrition; taking it together with mallow leads to fluid retention; taking it together with bamboo shoots leads to abdominal mass and heavy limbs unable to move. Children may suffer from decayed teeth and pinworms if taking it excessively.

榅桲不可多食，损齿伤筋。

Excessive taking of quince damages the teeth and sinews.

松子多食，发热毒。

Excessive taking of pine nuts causes heat toxin.

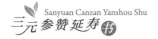
奈子多食，胪胀，不益人，病人尤甚。

Excessive taking of Naizi（a kind of apple）leads to abdominal distension, which is harmful to health, especially for patients.

胡桃，平，多食，利小便，脱人眉，动风，动痰，恶心呕吐。酒同食过多，咯血。

Walnut is mild in property. Excessive taking of it can promote urination, lead to loss of eyebrows, arouse internal wind and phlegm, cause nausea and vomiting.Taking it together with wine leads to hemoptysis.

五月食未成果核，发痈疖寒热。

Taking the unripe fruits in May causes carbuncle and furuncle, chills and fever.

秋夏果落地，恶虫缘，食之患九漏。

Taking the fallen fruits on the ground climbed by poisonous insect in summer and autumn may lead to nine kinds of fistulas.

一切果核双仁害人。

All fruits with double kernels are harmful to health.

生果停留多日，有损处，食之伤人。

Taking the raw fruits with scars which are kept for several days is harmful to health.

治诸果毒，烧猪骨过为末，水服方寸匕。

To treat the toxin of fruits, burn and grind the bones of pig into powder, take a square-inch-spoon of it with water.

米谷

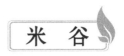

Grains

粳米，生者冷，燔者热，生不益脾，过熟则佳。苍耳同食，卒心痛；马肉同食，发痼疾。

The raw polished round-grained rice is cold in property, while the baked one is heat in property. The raw one is harmful to the spleen and the cooked one is beneficial to health. Taking it together with cocklebur leads to sudden precordial pain and taking it together with horse meat arouses chronic disease.

稻米，糯米也。妊娠与杂肉食之，不利其子，生寸白。久食身软，缓筋故也。性寒，壅经络气，使人四肢不收，昏闷多睡，发风动气，可少食。

Paddy rice is a kind of glutinous rice. Taking it together with various kinds of meat is harmful for the pregnant woman which may produce pinworms. Taking it for a long time can lead to weakness due to the lassitude of sinews induced. It is cold in property and can lead to qi stagnation of the meridians, spasm of the limbs，fainting and somnolence, disturbance of wind and qi in the body, thus people should control the amount when taking it.

秫米，似黍而小，亦可造酒。动风，不可常食。

Sorghum, which resembles millet but smaller than it, can be used to make wine. It can disturb wind in the body and ought not to be taken often.

黍米，发宿疾，久食昏五脏，好睡。小儿食，不能行，缓人筋骨，绝血脉。白黍久食，多热，令人烦。赤黍不可合蜜，惟可作糜。不可为饭，黏着难解。

Millet can arouse the abiding disease and long-time taking of it can damage the five zang-organs and lead to somnolence. The children who take it can not walk freely due to its action of weakening sinews and bones and stagnating vessels. Long-time taking of white millet causes vexation due to heat. Red millet should not be taken together with honey but can be made into porridge. It ought not to be taken for meal since it is too sticky.

五种黍米，合葵食之，成痼疾。藏脯于中，食之闭气。肺病者，宜此。

Taking the five kinds of millet together with mallow can lead to chronic disease. Taking it together with dried meat leads to suffocation, which is just the reason for lung diseases.

生米戏食，久为米瘕，肌瘦如劳，缺米则口吐清水。

Taking the raw rice for fun for a long term leads to conglomeration and

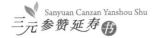

fatigue. Clear water would be spewed up if no rice is taken in.

饴糖进食，健胃，多食则动脾风。

Taking the proper amount of sugar improves appetite and invigorates the stomach, while excessive taking of it can lead to convulsive malaria.

麦占四时，秋种夏收。西北多霜雪，面无毒；南方少雪，有毒。

The whole growing process of wheat spans the four seasons, planted in autumn and harvested in the next summer. The flour produced in the northwest is not toxic since it snows and frosts often here. While flour produced in the south is toxic since it seldom snows.

小麦，性壅热，小动风气。治面后觉中毒，以酒咽汉椒三五粒，不为疾。

Wheat is heat in property and is prone to cause stagnation, which can disturb slightly the wind and qi of the body. If one feels poisoned during the preparation of wheat, try to swallow three to five pieces of Chinese pepper with wine and it will relieve it.

大麦，久食宜人，带生则冷，损人。

Barley is suitable for long-term taking and it benefits health, while the raw barley is cold in property and harmful for health.

麦蘖，久食消肾，不可多。

Taking germinated wheat for a long time damages the kidney, thus the amount should be controlled.

穬麦，西川多种，山东河北人，正月方种。先患冷气，人不宜食。

Kuangmai, a kind of wheat with arista, is widely planted in Xichuan. In Shandong and Hebei province, it is planted in January according to the lunar calendar. It may bring cold to the body, thus it is not suitable to be taken as food.

荞麦，性寒，难消。久食动风，头眩。和猪肉食八九次，患热风，脱眉须。

Buckwheat is cold in property and hard to digest. Long-time taking of it may lead to disturbance of internal wind and dizziness. If taking it together with pork for eight or nine times, it may cause syndrome of heat wind and the falling of eyebrow and beard.

粟米食后，勿食杏仁，令人吐泻。

Do not take almonds after taking corn, otherwise it may cause vomiting and diarrhea.

稷米，穄也，发三十六种病，八谷之中最为下。不可同川附子服。

Husked millet, also called prosomillet, can cause thirty six kinds of diseases, which ranks the lowest among the eight kinds of grains. It is forbidden to be taken together with Chuanfuzi [川附子, Monkshood-tuber,

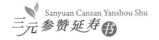

Radix Aconiti Lateralis Preparata〕.

陈廪粟米、秔米，陈者，性皆冷，频食之，自利。藏脯腊于中，满三月久，不知而食之，害人。

Stale corn and rice that have been stored for a long time are cold in property and can lead to diarrhea if taking frequently. Taking the dried meat which has been kept in the stale rice for three months is harmful to health.

绿豆治病，则皮不可去，去皮食少壅气。

If the mung beans are used to treat diseases, then the skin can not be removed. Taking it with the skin removed can avoid qi stagnation.

赤小豆，行小便，久食虚人，令人黑瘦枯燥。能逐津液，身体重。

The red beans can promote urination, while taking them for a long term leads to weakness, darkened skin, emaciation and dryness. It can also remove fluid retention and heaviness sensation of the body.

青小豆，一名胡豆，合鲤鱼鲊食之，肝黄，五年成干消。

Green beans, also called lima beans, if pickled together with carps, can lead to jaundice and consumptive thirst in five years.

赤白豆，合鱼鲊食之成消渴。

If the red white beans are pickled together with carps, they can lead to consumptive thirst.

黑白黄褐豆、大小豆，作豉极冷，黄卷及酱皆平，多食体重。服大豆末者，忌猪肉。炒豆与一岁以上十岁以下食之，即啖猪肉，久当拥气死人。有好食豆腐，中毒，不能治。更医至中途，遇作腐人家相争，因问，妻误将莱菔汤置锅中，腐更不成。医得其说，以莱菔汤下药而愈。莱菔，即萝卜也。

Beans of different colors such as black, white, yellow or brown beans and of different sizes, are all cold in property if they are fermented. The germinated and sauced soybean are mild in property, while taking an excessive amount of them leads to increased weight. The powder of the soybeans is incompatible with pork. If children who are above one but below ten years old take the stir-fried soybeans together with pork for long, it may lead to qi stagnation or even death. Once a person who liked to take bean-curd and was poisoned severely went to see doctor for treatment. On his way to another doctor, he met a family that made bean-curd in quarrel. He asked the reason and found out that the wife mistakenly put the soup of radish into the bean-curd pot, resulting in the failure of bean-curd formation. He told this to the doctor and the doctor prescribed radish soup for him and cured his poison. Radish is actually turnip.

酱当是豆为者。今以面麦为者，食之多杀药力。

The sauce should be made from soybeans. Presently, it is mostly made from flour, which reduces the effect of medicines if taking much.

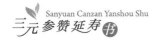
夫子云：不得其酱不食，故五脏悦而爱之，此亦安乐之端。

The Confucius said, "Food should only be taken together with its corresponding sauce with proper flavor to conform with the five zang-organs, which is also the origin of health and happiness."

脂麻炒熟，乘热压出生油，但可点。再煎炼方，方谓熟油，可食。

Stir-fry the sesame and crush it to produce raw oil when hot, which can only be used to light lamp. Fry and refine it again and then the cooked oil is produced, which is edible.

油，发冷疾，滑骨髓，困脾脏，经宿即动气。牙齿脾疾人，宜陈油，饮食须逐日熬熟。

Oil can cause cold diseases, make the marrow smooth, and encumber the spleen. It disorders qi if taking the oil kept for a night. Those with diseases of the teeth and the spleen should not take the stale oil but the newly cooked oil every day.

黑脂麻炒食之，不生风疾，风人日食之，则步履端正，语言不蹇。

Taking baked black sesames can protect people from suffering diseases like apoplexy. Stroke patients who take black sesames everyday are able to walk with firm and steady steps and talk fluently.

白脂麻，生则寒，炒则无发霍乱，抽人。又别有胡麻，味苦。乃苣胜也，不可为补益用。乌麻最益人。

The raw white sesames are cold in property, and the baked ones can protect people from suffering from cholera and spasm. There is also flax, bitter in taste, being another kind of sesamum indicum, which can not be used as tonic. Black sesames are the most beneficial for health.

胡麻，一名苣胜，服之不老，耐风湿，补衰老。九蒸九曝，末之，以枣膏丸服之，治白发还黑。补五内，益气力，长肌肉，填骨髓脑，坚筋骨。久服轻身不老，明耳目，耐饥渴，延年。

Flax, also named Jusheng, can help to keep people young, improve body resistence to rheumatism and slow aging. Steam and expose it in the sun for nine times, pound it into powder, mix it with date paste, and make them into pills. They can turn white hair black, nourish the five zang-organs, benefit the strength and muscle, strengthen the marrow and the brain, fortify the tendon and bone. Long time taking of it may keep one young and healthy, improve vision and hearing, get better resistence against hunger and thirst, and prolong longevity.

白麻油与乳母食，其孩子永不生病。治饮食逐日熬熟，用经宿即动气，有牙齿并脾胃疾人，切不可吃。

The baby fed by wet nurse taking white sesame oil as food will hardly get ill. When used as food, it should be cooked and taken within a day instead of overnight. Otherwise it may disturb qi. It should not be taken for those with diseases involving teeth, spleen and stomach.

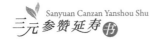
大麻仁，不宜多食，损血脉，滑精气，痿阳气，妇人多食，发带疾。以五升同葱一握捣和，浸三日，去滓沐发，令白发不生。研取汁，煎三十余沸收之，常取汁和羹兼煮粥，食之，去一切五脏气。

Hemp kernel should not be taken excessively, otherwise it may damage the blood and vessels, cause spontaneous seminal emission, impair yang, and lead to leukorrhea for women. Take 5 Sheng of it, smash it together with a handful of green onion, immerse them for 3 days, filter the dregs and get the juice to wash hair. This can prevent the production of white hair. Grind the hemp kernel to get the juice, boil it 30 times, take some to cook together with soup or porridge, this can dispel pathogenic factors in the five zang-organs.

菜 蔬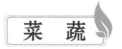

Vegetables

葵，为五菜主，秋种。早者至春作子，名冬葵。其心有毒，伤人。性冷，熟食之亦令热闷，甚动风气。葵冻者，生食之，动五种留饮，甚则吐水。和鲤鱼食之，害人。四季勿食生葵，不化，发人一切宿疾。百药忌食之，发狂犬咬。

Curled mallow is the top among the five main vegetables. It is planted in autumn and bears seeds from early spring to mid-spring, also known as malva crispa. The heart of it is toxic and is harmful to health. It is cold in property, and the cooked ones can also lead to heat stagnation and wind diseases. Taking the frozen curled mallow can cause five kinds of fluid retention and even water-spitting. Taking it together with carps is harmful to health. The raw ones are not suitable to take in the four seasons since they are hard to be digested and can cause abiding ailment. Do not take it together with all medicinals, otherwise it may lead to rabies.

吴葵，一名蜀葵，不可久食，钝人志性。被狗咬戒食，误食之，

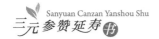
永不瘥。

Wukui, also called hollyhock, is not suitable for long-term taking, which can slow down one's action and thinking. It is forbidden to take it when bitten by dog. If taking it mistakenly, one may never recover from diseases.

戎葵，并鸟肉食，无颜色。

Taking hollyhock together with bird meat worsens the complexion.

生葱，食之即啖蜜，下痢。食烧葱啖蜜，拥气，死。杂白犬肉食之，九窍出血，患气者多发，气上充人，五脏闭绝，虚人胃，开骨节。正月食之，生面上游风。大抵功在发汗，多则昏人神。

Taking honey immediately after raw scallion causes dysentery. Taking honey immediately after cooked scallion leads to qi stagnation and even death. Taking the scallion together with the meat of white dogs leads to bleeding of the nine orifices, which often occurs in patients with qi diseases resulting in counter-flow of qi, stagnation of the five zang-organs, stomach deficiency and lassitude of joints. Taking it in the first month of the lunar year can cause urticaria on the face. Its major function is to promote sweating and the excessive taking of it may cause dizziness.

胡葱，多食伤神，损性，多忘，损目发痼疾。狐臭、䘌齿人食之甚。青鱼合食，生虫。

Excessive taking of shallot damages spirit and constitution, leads to amnesia, impairs eyesight and induces abiding ailment. Those suffering from bromhidrosis or decayed teeth should not take it since it may worsen their diseases. Taking it together with black carp leads to parasitic diseases.

韭，俗呼草钟乳，病人可食。然多食昏神暗目，酒后尤忌。不可与蜜同食。未出土为韭黄，不益人，滞气。花，动风。过清明勿食，不利病人，心腹痼疾者加剧。

Leeks, which is also called Caozhongru, are suitable for patients to take. Excessive taking of it leads to dizziness and blurred vision, which should be forbidden to take after drinking in particular. It can not be taken together with honey. The leek whose root is still below the ground is called chive, which is not beneficial for health and can lead to qi stagnation. Its flowers disturb internal wind in the body. It should not be taken after Qingming festival for its negative effect on patients and worsening effect on those with chronic diseases involving the heart and abdomen.

霜韭不可食，动宿饮，必吐水。五月食之，损人滋味，乏气力。不可共牛肉食，成瘕。热病后十日，不可食，发困。葱亦不宜。

Frost leeks are not edible because they can induce abiding fluid retention and lead to water-spitting. Taking leeks in May can damage the sense of taste and lead to flaccidity. It should not be taken together with beef, which can cause abdominal mass. It should not be taken until ten days after heat syndrome, which can cause drowsiness. The same is true with scallion.

薤，肥健人。生食，引涕唾。与牛肉食，作瘕。四月勿食薤。三冬至食，

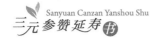
多涕唾。

Chinese Chive can make people healthy and strong. Taking the raw ones causes tears and saliva and taking it together with beef leads to abdominal mass. It should not be taken in April. Taking much of it in winter leads to production of tears and saliva.

葫，大蒜也。久食伤肝损目，弱阳。煮以合青鱼鲊发黄，作齑，啖鲙伐命。惟生食，不中煮。暑毒，烂嚼下咽即和。仍禁冷水。四月、八月，食之伤神，损胆气，喘悸气急，腹内生疮，肠肿成疝瘕。多食葫行房，伤肝，面无光。北方人禀厚者，食惯，病少。

Garlic is also called Hu. Long-time taking of it damages the liver and vision, causes weak potency of men. Boiling it together with pickled black carps makes its color brown. It is deadly to take the chopped garlic and Chinese herring together. It is better to be taken raw without boiling. Chew and swallow it and then the summer heatstroke can be relieved. It is forbidden to drink cold water during this period. Taking it in April or August damages the spirit, the gallbladder qi and leads to asthma, palpitation, shortness of breath, abdominal sores, abdominal mass and hernia due to swelling of the intestines. Taking garlic before having sexual activity damages the liver and leads to poor complexion. The northerners with good constitution are accustomed to taking it, which helps to prevent diseases.

小蒜不可常食，食而啖生鱼，夺气，阴核疼欲死。三月勿食，伤志。时病瘥后，与一切食，竟入房，病发必死。

The rocambole is not appropriate for taking frequently. Taking it together with raw fish consumes qi and leads to acute genital pain. Taking it in March impairs the mentality. After short recovery from seasonal diseases, one may still die if having sexual activity after taking rocambole with other food.

胡荽，荞子也。久食令人多忘，狐臭、口气、䘌齿、脚气加剧。根发痼疾。

Coriander is also called Qiaozi. Long-time taking of it leads to amnesia, bromhidrosis, smelly breath, decayed teeth and aggravation of beriberi. Taking the root of it induces the abiding ailment.

蓼子，是水浸令生芽而食之者。多食令人吐水，损阳少精，心痛寒热，损骨髓。二月食之，伤肾。和生鱼食，夺阴气，核子痛，欲死。

Polygonum is usually soaked in water to sprout for people to eat. Excessive taking of it induces water-spitting, damages yang and essence of the body, leads to pain of the heart and chills and fever, impairs the marrow. Taking it in February damages the kidney and taking it together with raw fish damages yin and leads to severe pain of vulva.

萱草，一名忘忧，嫩时取以为蔬。食之动风，令人昏昏然，终日如醉，因得其名。

Daylily, which is also called Wang You（refers to forgetting sorrow）, can be taken as vegetables when it is tender. It may disturb internal wind

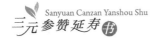

and make people drowsy like being drunk all day, which is the reason for its being called Wang You.

菘，发诸风冷。有热人食之，不发病，性冷也。

Chinese cabbage can cause wind and cold syndrome. It is cold in property so it is safe for people with heat syndrome to take.

芥，多食动风气，发丹石。与兔肉同食，成恶病。

Mustard can disturb internal wind and cause the toxin of elixir if taking excessively. Taking it together with the meat of rabbit causes malignant diseases.

芜青，蔓青也。根不可多食，令气胀。子作油涂头，发黑。

Turnip is also called Man Qing. Its root can not be taken excessively, which may cause flatulence. To smear the oil extracted from its seeds on hair can make the hair black and bright.

莱菔即萝卜，力弱人不宜多食，生者渗人血。

Lai Fu is actually radish, which is not suitable for people with weak constitution to take. The raw ones can cause blood extravasation.

生青菜，时病瘥后食之，手足青肿。

To take the raw Chinese cabbage after recovering from the seasonal diseases may lead to bruise and swelling of the hands and feet.

一切菜，五月五日勿食之，变百病。

It is forbidden to take any vegetable in May the fifth, which may cause various diseases.

一切菜，熟煮热食之。凡澹流滴着者，有毒。

All vegetables should be taken when cooked and heated. They are toxic if mixed with water from eaves or chopsticks.

十月被霜菜，食者面无光，目涩，腰疼，心疟。发时，足十指爪青，萎困。

To take the vegetables frosted in October may lead to poor complexion, dry eyes, low back pain, and heart malaria, which is manifested with symptoms of cyanotic nails of the feet, flaccidity and drowsiness.

荠菜，不宜面同食，令人督闷发病，凡用甘草皆忌此。

Shepherd's purse should not be taken together with flour, which may lead to dizziness, distress and other diseases. This taboo is also applicable to the usage of Gancao［甘草, Liquorice Root, Radix Glycyrrhizae］.

苋菜多食动气，烦闷，冷中损腹。共蕨及鳖食，生瘕。

Taking an excessive amount of edible amaranth disturbs internal qi, causes vexation and cold in the middle, and impairs the abdomen. Taking it together with fern and turtle meat leads to abdominal mass.

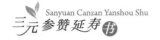

堇菜不宜多食，令人身重，多肿，只可一二顿。

Taking an excessive amount of violet leads to heaviness and swelling of the body. Thus it can only be taken once or twice

芸薹菜，患腰脚人多食加剧。损阳气，发口疮，齿痛，生虫。狐臭人忌之。

Taking an excessive amount of winter rape can aggravate the disease involving the waist and legs. It damages yang qi, causes aphtha, toothache and parasitic diseases. Those suffering from body odor should not take it.

鹿角菜，久食发宿疾，损经络，少颜色。

Long-time taking of pelvetia silquosa induces abiding ailment, damages the meridians and worsens complexion.

菠薐菜，北人食肉面即平，南人食鱼米即冷。多食，冷大小肠。久食，脚软腰痛。

Spinach is mild for Northerners who take meat and flour more, while cold for Southerners who take fish and rice more. Excessive taking of it can cause cold in the large intestine and small intestine. Taking it for a long time leads to pedal flaccidity and pain in the waist.

莼菜，多食性滑发痔，引疫气，上有水银故也。七月蜡虫着上，令霍乱，勿食之。

Water shield is lubricant in property and excessive taking of it leads to haemorrhoids and pestilent disease for the mercury on it. Do not take it in July for the mealybug clung on it, which may lead to cholera.

芹菜生高田者，宜人。黑滑地名水芹，赤色者害人，性寒，和醋食之损齿。

Celery planted in high-lying fields benefits health. Those that planted in dark marsh are called water celery, among which the red ones are cold in property and harmful to health. Taking it together with vinegar damages the teeth.

春秋，龙带精入芹中，偶食之，手青肚满，痛不可忍，服砂糖三二斤，吐出蚰蜒，便愈。

In spring and autumn, the sperm of the lizard might be hidden in celery, which can cause purplish hands, stomach distention and unbearable pain if taken incidentally. It can be cured by taking two to three Jin of sugar to induce the spitting of the scorpion lizard.

苦荬，夏月食之以益心，蚕妇忌食之。

Taking bitter endive during summer benefits the heart. It is forbidden for women who raise silkworms to take since its smell can impair the larva of the silkworms.

莴苣，冷，久食昏人目。白莴苣，冷气人食之，腹冷。产后不可食，寒中。共饴食，生虫。苦苣不可与蜜同食。

Lettuce is cold in property and long-term taking of it blurs vision. The

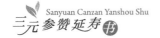

white ones are not suitable for people with cold syndrome since they bring more cold to the abdomen. It is not suitable for women to take after delivery for its damage to the middle. Taking it together with sugar leads to parasitic diseases. The bitter lettuce ought not to be taken together with honey.

莙荙，多食动气，冷气人食之，必破腹。

Taking an excessive amount of chard disturbs qi in the body. It can lead to diarrhea if being taken by those with cold syndrome.

苜蓿利大小肠。蜜食下痢，多食瘦人。

Alfalfa can disinhibit the large and small intestines. Taking it together with honey leads to dysentery and excessive taking of it causes emaciation.

蕨，久食脚弱无力，弱阳，眼暗多睡，鼻塞，发落。小儿食之，不行。冷气食之，腹胀。生食成蛇瘕。

Taking fern for a long time leads to flaccidity and weakness of the feet, diminished yang, blurred vision, drowsiness, stuffy nose and losing of hair. Children who take it may suffer from inability to walk. If those with cold syndrome take it, they may suffer from abdominal distention. If taken raw, it may lead to abdominal mass in the form of snakes.

郄鉴镇丹徒出猎，有甲士折一枚食之，觉心淡淡成疾，后吐一小蛇，悬屋前，渐成干蕨，信不可生食蕨也。

Once there were people in the town of Qiejian town going hunting. One warrior took a piece of fern and swallowed it. Later he felt uncomfortable in the heart and spit out something like a small snake, which was dried into fern after hanging in front of the house for some time. Thus it was believed that fern could not be taken raw.

茄，至冷，五劳不可多食，发疮损人，动气发痼疾。熟者少食无忧患。冷人不可食。秋后食之损目。

Eggplant is severely cold in property and is not appropriate to take for people with five kinds of consumptive diseases. Otherwise, it may lead to sores, impair health, disturb qi and induce abiding ailment. It is suitable to take after being cooked in proper amount. It is not suitable for people with cold syndrome to take. Taking it after autumn damages the eyes.

黄瓜，本名胡瓜，不益人。患脚气虚肿者，毒永不除。

Cucumber, originally named Hu Gua, is not beneficial for health. Those who suffer from beriberi and puffiness should not take it, otherwise their diseases may never be cured.

越瓜色白，动气发疮，脚弱，不益小儿。时病后勿食。与乳酪鲊及空心食，心痛。

Snake melon is white in color, which may disturb qi, induce sores and flaccidity of the feet. It is not suitable for children and those who have just recovered from seasonal diseases to take. Taking it together with pickled cheese or on empty stomach leads to heartache.

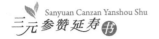

青瓜，令人多忘。

Green cucumber may lead to forgetfulness.

冬瓜多食，阴湿生疮，发黄疸。九月勿食。被霜瓜，向冬发血寒热，反恶。病初食，吐食竟，心下停水，或为翻胃。有冷者，食之瘦。瓜能暗人眼，尤不宜老人。中其毒，至秋为疟痢。一切瓜，苦者有毒。两蒂两鼻者，害人。

Excessive taking of white gourd leads to sores due to dampness and jaundice. It should not be taken in September. Taking the frosted gourds leads to blood cold and heat syndrome and induces malignant diseases. Taking it at the onset of disease leads to vomiting, fluid retention below the heart or gastric disorder with nausea. Those with cold syndrome may suffer from emaciation if taking it. It can also cause blurred vision, which is especially not suitable for the old to take. It may lead to malarial dysentery in autumn if taking the toxic ones. All the melons with bitter taste are toxic. Melons with two pedicles are harmful to health.

瓠子，冷气人食之病甚，大耗食。患脚气虚肿人食之，毒永不除。

Bottle gourd aggravates the condition of people with cold syndrome and it may lead to consumption of essence. Those who suffer from beriberi and deficient swelling are hard to be cured of the toxicity.

葫芦，多食令人吐。

Excessive taking of gourd can lead to vomiting.

芋，一名土芝，有紫有白。冬月食，不发病，他月不可食。

Taro, also called Tu Zhi, is white or purple in color. It is suitable to be taken during the months in winter while it ought not to be taken in other months.

薯蓣，亦有紫白，颇胜芋。有小而名山药者佳。

Chinese yam is purple or white in color too, which is much better in quality than taroes. The smaller ones called Shan Yao are of good quality.

蒟蒻，冷气人少食之。

Konnyaku is not suitable for people with cold syndrome to take.

曾有患瘵，自谓无生，是物不忌，邻家修蒟蒻，求食之，美，遂多食，竟愈。有病腮痈者数人，余教多食此而愈。

Once there was a patient suffering from tuberculosis could see no hope for his recovery, so he didn't restrain himself at all in diet. When he saw his neighbor trimming Konnyaku, he asked for some to eat and found it delicious. Then he ate a lot and surprisingly, he recovered from his disease. I once told several patients suffering from parotid carbuncle to take much Konnyaku and they all healed finally.

甜瓜多食，令人阴下痒湿生疮，发黄疸病。凡瓜入水沉者，食之得冷气，终身不瘥。

Muskmelon, if taken excessively, may lead to itchiness and dampness of

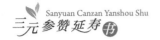

external genitalia, sore, and jaundice. Those that sink in the water may lead to cold syndrome which is hard to cure for the lifetime.

上床萝卜下床姜。盖夜间萝卜消宿食，早起姜能开胃也。

Take some radish when one gets down to sleep and some ginger when one gets up. The reason is that radish can help to relieve food retention during nighttime and ginger can help to improve appetite in the morning.

萝卜和羊肉食，下五脏一切气，令人肥白。如无羊肉，诸鱼肉皆得用也。久服涩肠卫，令人发早白。

Radish, if taken together with mutton, can conduct qi of the five zang-organs downward and keep one strong and lustrous. If there is no mutton available, it can be taken together with fish meat. Long time taking of it can astring the intestines and result in white hair at an early age.

牛蒡，通十二经脉，洗五脏拥气，可常菜食。

Burdock has the function of dredging the channels and removing stagnation of the five zang-organs, so it can be taken frequently.

蔊菜细切，以生蜜洗或略煎，吃之爽口，妙，能消宿食。多食发痼疾。昆布多食令人瘦。

Rorippa indica, if taken after mixing with raw honey or fried slightly after being sliced thinly, is tasty and refreshing, with the function of treating indigestion. If taken excessively, it may induce abiding ailment. Kelp, if taken excessively, may lead to emaciation.

紫菜多食，令人腹痛，发气吐白沫，饮少热醋解。

Nori, if taken excessively, can result in abdominal pain, cause counterflow of qi with foaming at the mouth, which can be relieved by drinking a little hot vinegar.

决明叶，明目轻身，利五脏，作菜食之良。子主肝家热，每日取一匙，将去土，空腹吞之，百日后夜见字。

Cassia leaf, with the function of improving eyesight, keeping the physique young and benefiting the five zang-organs, is good to be taken as vegetable. Cassia seed is indicated for removing heat in the liver. Swallow one spoon of it each day on empty stomach after cleaning it, and one is capable of reading clearly at night.

干苔，发诸疮疥，下一切丹石，杀诸药毒。不可多食，令人动血气。

Fried moss can induce various sores and scabies, reduce the effect of taking the elixir and remove toxicity of various medicinals. It should not be taken excessively, otherwise it may disturb blood and qi of the body.

茭白，不可合生菜食之。多食发气并弱阳，不可杂蜜食之，发痼疾。主心胸中浮热动气。不中食，发冷，滋牙齿，伤阳道，不食为妙。

Water bamboo is forbidden to be taken together with lettuce. Excessive

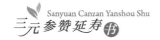

taking of it may disturb qi and impair yang of the body. It should not be taken together with honey, otherwise it may lead to abiding ailment. It is indicated for floating heat and disturbed qi in the chest. It is better not to take it when one is suffering from poor appetite, chills, bared teeth and impaired yang.

苦笋，主不睡，去面目并舌下热黄消渴。明目，解热毒，除热气，健人。

Bitter bamboo shoot is indicated for difficulty in falling asleep, heat in the face, the eyes and the tongue, consumptive thirst. It can improve eyesight, relieve heat toxin, expel heat pathogen and benefit health.

笋箭，笋新者稍可食，陈者不可食。

Tips of bamboo shoots are edible when they are tender and inedible when they are overgrown.

淡竹笋，虽口美，发背闷、脚气。

Dried bamboo shoot, though tasty, can lead to back distress and beriberi.

笋以薄荷叶数片同煮，即无食味。

The acerbity of bamboo shoot can be removed by boiling it together with several mint leaves.

诸笋煮二三日不烂，脾难克化，脾病者，不宜吃。

Bamboo shoot that can not be cooked thoroughly in 2 or 3 days is not suitable to be taken as food for those with spleen disorder, as it is hard to be transported and transformed by spleen.

生姜，九月九日勿食之，伤神损寿。干姜，妊多食内消。

Fresh ginger, if taken on the ninth in September, damages the spirit and shortens the lifespan. Dried ginger, if taken much by pregnant women, causes internal consumptive disease.

椿芽，多食神昏。

Excessive taking of Chinese toon sprout causes unconsciousness.

榆仁，多食发热、心痛。

Excessive taking of elm kernel leads to fever and heartache.

菌，地生为菌，木生为檽、为木耳、为蕈。新蕈有毛者、下无纹者、夜有光者、煮不熟者、欲烂无虫者、煮讫照人无影者、春夏有恶虫毒蛇经过者，皆杀人。误食毒菌，往往笑不止而死。惟掘地为坎，投水搅，取清者饮之。

Fungus refers to the field-born plant, while the one growing on trees is called agaric, edible tree fungus or mushroom. It is deadly to take these kinds of mushrooms like fresh ones with hair, ones with no lines in the bottom, ones giving out light at night, ones hard to cook, rotten ones but without insects on, ones unable to reflect image after being cooked, and ones crawled on by poisonous insects or snakes in spring and summer. Taking poisonous

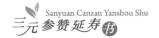

fungus by mistake may lead to death due to endless laughing. The only way to treat it is to dig a pit, fill it with water, stir and wait till the water is clear, and then drink the water.

木菌，楮、槐、榆、柳、桑五木之耳，可食。冬春无毒。木耳亦不宜多食，如前所云者皆杀人。又：赤色仰面不覆者，及生野田中者，皆毒。又：发冷风气痔，多睡，无力。

Timber fungi, including the ear of the Broussonetia papyrifera, Sophora japonica, elm, willow and mulberry, are edible. They are nontoxic if collected in winter and spring. They should not be taken excessively and just as mentioned above, they are deadly to take in certain conditions. It is also said that the red uncurled ones and those growing in wild are toxic. It is also said that they may lead to internal cold and wind, hemorrhoids, somnolence, and flaccidity.

甘露子不宜生食，不可多食，生寸白虫，与诸鱼同食，病生反胃。

Chinese artichoke ought not to be taken raw or excessively, otherwise it may lead to pinworm. Taking it together with fishes leads to gastric disorder with nausea.

茱萸，六七月食之伤神气。

Cornel may damage spirit and vitality if taken in June or July.

茼蒿多食，气满。

Excessive taking of crowndaisy leads to qi stagnation.

莳萝根，曾有食者杀人。

Dill root is said to have caused death of the people who took it.

蔓菁，菜中之最益人者，常食之，通中益气，令人肥健。

Turnip, the most beneficial vegetable for health, is appropriate for frequent taking with the function of regulating qi circulation and invigorating the body health.

兰香不可多食，壅关节，涩荣卫，令人血脉不行，又动风，发脚气。

Basil should not be taken excessively for it may stagnate the joints, the nutrient and defensive qi, hinder the circulation of blood and vessel, disturb internal wind and induce beriberi.

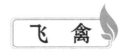

Fowls

鸡，黄者宜老人，乌者暖血，产妇宜之。具五色，食者必狂。六指玄鸡、白头家鸡，及野禽生子有八字文，及死不伸足，害人。

The yellow-colored chicken is suitable for the elderly to take and the black-colored one is suitable for lying-in women to take. The five-colored chicken may lead to mania for people who take it. It is deadly to take black chickens with six claws, white-headed domestic chickens, wild-born chickens with splayed patterns on their bodies, and those with curled claws after death.

乌鸡合鲤鱼食，生痈疽。

Taking silkie and carp together may result in ulcer and carbuncle.

丙午日食鸡肉，主丈夫烧死，目盲，女人血死，妄见。

Taking chickens on the day of Bingwu may lead to man burning to death and turning blind, woman dying from blood diseases and bearing false senses.

《千金方》载：四月勿食暴鸡肉，作疽、液漏，男女虚劳、乏气。八月食之伤神气。妊妇多食，子患诸虫。

Qian Jin Fang（《千金方》, *Valuable Prescriptions worth Thousand Gold*）says: In April, it is forbidden to take pestilent chicken, which may cause subcutaneous ulcer, liquorrhea, consumptive diseases and qi deficiency for both men and women. Taking it in August damages qi and spirit. Excessive taking of it for pregnant women may lead to parasitic diseases of the fetus.

妊食鸡子，多令子失音。

Taking eggs during pregnancy may cause dumbness of the baby.

鸡子动风、动气，合鳖肉食害人；合犬肝、犬肉食泄利害人；合鱼汁内成心瘕；合獭肉及野鸡共家鸡肉合食之，成遁尸，尸鬼缠身，四肢百节疼痛。

Eggs can disturb the internal wind and qi in the body, and taking it together with turtle meat is harmful to health; taking it together with the liver or meat of dogs leads to diarrhea; taking it together with fish or meat extract leads to abdominal mass of the heart; taking it together with the meat of otter, pheasant or chicken leads to a kind of acute disease called Dunshi in Chinese with symptoms of abdominal distention, stabbing pain of the heart and asthma, feeling like being held up by ghosts and featured with pain in limbs and joints.

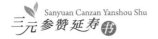

鸡子白，合胡荽、葱、蒜食，短气；合生葱、犬肉食，谷道流血。

Egg white, if taken together with coriandrum, scallion and garlic, may lead to shortness of breath; if taken together with green onion and dog meat, may lead to bleeding in the esophagus.

疹，食鸡、鸭子，眼翳。

Taking chicken or duck eggs when suffering from rash leads to corneal opacity.

鸡，过宿收不密，蜈蚣必集其中，不再煮而食之，为害非轻。

The chicken, if not properly stored and healed at night, is sure to attract centipedes coming inside it, which can bring on damage to health if taking without cooking again the next day.

鸡并子不可合李子食之。老鸡能呼人姓名，杀之则止。

Chicken and egg should not be taken together with plum. The old chicken may know how to call a person's name, which can be ended by killling it.

鸡有四距重翼者，龙也，杀之震死。

The chicken with 4 spurs and 2 wings is actually dragon, which may lead to death if killing it.

乌鸡最暖，可补血，妇人可食。

Silkie chicken has the function of warming and nourishing blood, which is suitable for women to take.

阉鸡善啼，内毒。

Capon is good at crowing and it is toxic inside.

踏鸡子壳令人得白瘢风。半夜鸡啼则有忧事。

Stepping on egg shells may lead to vitiligo. If chicken crows at night, this may indicate the possible happening of sorrow.

鸡生子皆雄者必有喜事。

If all the eggs hatched out are male, this is an indication of happy event.

雉，离禽也。损多益少，久食瘦人，春夏多食有毒。九十至十一月稍补，他月发痔及疮疥。八月忌之。益人神气。丙午日不可食，明主于火也。四月勿食，气逆。和胡桃、菌子同食，下血，有痼疾者不宜。和荞麦面食，生肥虫。卵不与葱同食，生寸白。

The pheasant is a kind of bird with glorious feathers, which brings less benefit and more damage to health. Long-time taking of it causes emaciation and excessive taking of it in spring and summer is toxic to health. It has the function of nourishing if taken from September to November but induces hemorrhoids, sores and scabies if taken in other months. It is forbidden to take in August. It is beneficial to spirit and vitality. It is forbidden to take

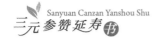
on the day of Bingwu because this day pertains to fire and the pheasant meat pertains to yang, which may easily lead to internal heat and wind. It is forbidden to take in April, otherwise it may cause counter-flow of qi. Taking it together with walnut and fungus causes discharge of blood. It is not suitable for people with chronic diseases. Taking it together with buckwheat brings on worm eggs and taking it together with scallion results in pinworms.

鹜，鸭也。六月勿食，益神气。黑鸭滑中，发冷痢。脚气人不可多食，有毒。妊娠多食，令子倒生。

Duck ought not to be taken in June. It has the function of benefiting spirit and vitality. Black duck can lubricate the middle and induce dysentery. Those suffering from beriberi should not take much of it for its toxicity. It may lead to reversed fetal position if taken much during pregnancy.

野鸭不可与胡桃、木耳同食。

Wild duck should not be taken together with walnuts and edible tree fungus.

《异苑》曰：章安有人元嘉中啖鸭肉成瘕，胸满面赤，不得饮食。医以秫米食之，须臾吐一鸭雏，遂瘥。此因内生所致，又食过而然。

Yi Yuan（《异苑》, *A Collection of Strange Stories*）says: During Yuan Jia years of the Northern and Southern Dynasty, a person in Zhangan suffered from abdominal mass, chest fullness, red complexion and poor appetite because he took much of duck. The doctor let him take some husked sorghum. Soon he spit out a duckling and then recovered. It is because the disease is caused by his taking raw duck meat excessively.

白鸭补虚，目白者杀人。鸭卵多食发疾冷气。

White duck can tonify deficiency and those with white eyes can be deadly to take. Excessive taking of duck eggs induces diseases involving cold syndrome.

老鸭善，嫩鸭毒。

Old duck is beneficial for health and young duck is harmful for health.

鸭子不可合蒜食之，又不可合李子、鳖肉食之。

Duck is contraindicated with garlic, plum and turtle meat.

野鸭九月已后，即中食，全胜家者，虽寒不动气。又身上生热疮，多年不好者，但多食之即瘥。

Wild duck is better than domestic duck to be taken after September, being cold in property but with no danger to disturb qi. Refractory and perennial herpes simplex can be cured by taking abundant wild duck.

白鹅肉性冷，多食霍乱，发痼疾。卵不可多食。苍鹅发疮脓。老鹅善，嫩鹅毒。鹅毛柔暖而性冷，选细毛夹以布帛，絮而为被，偏宜覆婴儿而辟惊痫也。

The meat of white goose is cold in property and excessive taking of it can lead to cholera and induce chronic diseases. Their eggs should not be

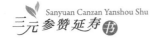

taken excessively. Taking the meat of gray-white-colored goose can cause sores and pus.

鹌鹑，四月已后，八月已前，不堪食。本草云：虾蟆化也。鹑，患痢人可煮食之，良。和生羹煮食泄痢，酥煎偏令下焦肥。与猪肝同食面生黑子。与菌同食发痔疾。

Quail is not suitable to take from April to August. *Ben Cao*（《本草》, *Classic of Materia Medica*）says: It is transformed from frogs. Quail can be boiled and taken by and beneficial for those suffering from dysentery. It can result in diarrhea if cooked together with raw soup and greasy lower energizer if fried crisply. Taking it together with pig liver leads to black spots on the face and taking it together with fungus leads to hemorrhoids.

鹧鸪，鸪不可与笋同食，令人腹胀。此鸟天地之神，每月取一只飨，至尊。自死者忌之。

Partridge, if taken together with bamboo shoot, may lead to abdominal distention. It is regarded as something like the God of heaven and earth. Taking one for dinner every month brings the supreme enjoyment. Do not take the naturally dead ones.

山鸡顿食发五痔。和荞麦食生疮。不与豉同食，杀人。卵不可与葱同食，生寸白。不可久食，令人疫。惊雉，一名山鸡，养之禳火灾。山鸡类也。

Berghaan may lead to five kinds of hemorrhoids if taken for every meal. If taken together with buckwheat, it leads to sores. If taken together with fermented soya beans, it leads to death. Its eggs, if taken together with green onion, lead to production of pinworms. If taken for a long time, it leads to pestilence. Primitive pheasant, also named berghaan, averts fire disaster. So do berghaans.

南唐相冯延巳，苦脑痛，久不减，太医吴延绍诰。庖人曰："相公平日多食鹧鸪、山鸡。" 吴曰："得之矣。" 投以甘草汤而愈。盖此禽多食乌头、半夏，有毒，以此解之。又《类编》：通判杨立之官南方，多食鹧鸪，生喉痈，脓血日夕不止。泗水杨吉老，令先啖生姜一斤，愈。盖以制半夏毒也。唐崔魏公，以多食竹鸡暴亡，梁新命捩生姜汁，折齿灌之，复活。亦此意也。

Feng Yansi, the prime minister of the Nantang dynasty, suffered from a severe headache which could not be relieved for a long time. Wu Yanshao, the imperial doctor, received the emperor's order and went to treat him. The chef said, "The prime minister is fond of taking partridges and pheasants as food in dinner." The doctor replied, "I know the reason for his disease." He treated the prime minister with Gancao Tang（Licorice Decoction）and cured his disease. It is because these fowls often feed on Wutou［乌头, the Rhizome of Chinese Monkshood, Aconitum］and Banxia［半夏, Pinellia Tuber, Rhizoma Pinelliae］, which are toxic and can be relieved by Gancao decoction. *Lei Bian*［《类编》, *Classics Arranged by Category*］says: Yang Lizhi, the governor of the state, was an official in the south who liked to take partridges. Once he suffered from throat abscess, and the pus and blood oozed endlessly. The famous doctor, Yang Jilao from Si Shui asked him to take one Jin of fresh ginger and then he recovered. The reason is that ginger can relieve the toxicity of Banxia［半夏, Pinellia Tuber, Rhizoma Pinelliae］. Cui Weigong of the Tang Dynasty died suddenly because he took too many bamboo partridges. Liang Xin asked the servant to grind some fresh ginger juice, pry open his mouth, and pour the juice in, then Cui Weigong came back to

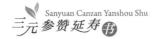

life. This is because of the same reason.

鸳鸯肉常食之患大风。夫妇不相和，煮鸳鸯肉食之，即时和顺相爱也。

Mandarin duck can lead to severe wind syndrome if taking frequently. The disharmony of married couple can be treated by taking boiled meat of mandarin duck. They will restore mutural love immediately.

雀肉不与李同食。合酱食妊娠所忌。不可合杂生肝食之。雀粪和老姜末蜜丸服之，令人肥白。

Sparrow is forbidden to be taken together with plum, to be taken together with sauce for pregnant women and to be taken together with raw liver. Mix sparrow manure and ginger powder with honey into pills. Take them and then one will become strong and have improved complexion.

鹁鸽虽益人，病者食之，多减药力。

Pigeon can benefit health, but it may reduce the efficacy of the medicine for patients.

雄鹊妇人不可食。烧毛纳水中，沉者是雄。

Male magpie is not suitable for women to take. The method to recognize the male magpie is to burn its feather and put it into water. If it sinks, then it is male magpie.

乌鸦肉涩不中食。鸦瘦，病嗽骨蒸者，可和五味腌炙食之。鸦眼睛，研，注人目中，令人见神鬼。

The meat of crow is puckery and unsuitable to be taken as food. Crow meat, picked and broiled with five kinds of flavors, can treat cough caused by hectic fever due to yin deficiency. Eyes of crow, if ground and dropped into the eyes, may produce ghost-like illusion.

燕肉，人不可食，入水必为蛟龙所害，食者损人神气。出《千金博物志》。

Meat of swallow ought not to be taken as food. Otherwise, one may be injured by dragon in water. It damages the spirit and vitality. This is recorded in *Qian Jin Bo Wu Zhi*（《千金博物志》, *Records of Natural Science Worth One Thousand Gold*）

雁肉勿食，损人神气。脂，可和豆黄末服，令人肥白。

The meat of wild goose is inedible as it impairs spirit and vitality. Mixing its fat with soy powder and taking it can make people strong and shiny.

孔雀毛入人眼即瞎。诸般死鸟皆不可食。

Peacock feather, if dropped in the eyes, results in blindness. All the dead birds are inedible.

杜鹃初鸣，先闻者主别离。学其声吐血。厕上闻者，不祥，作犬声

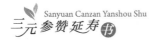
应之，吉。

The cuckoo's first chirp indicates separation for those who hear it firstly. Those who imitate its sound may spit blood. It's not auspicious to hear cuckoo singing above toilet, but it is propitious to imitate dog's bark to respond.

凡禽自死，口不闭者，杀人。

It is fatal to take the meat of naturally dead birds whose mouth is not closed after death.

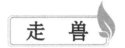

走 兽

Beasts

猪肉之用最多，然不宜人，食之暴肥，致风虚也。闭血脉，弱筋骨，虚人肌，病人，金疮者尤甚。食其肉饮酒，不可卧秫穰中。又白猪白蹄杂青者，不可食。猪肾理肾气，多食肾虚，久食少子。

Pork is taken frequently but it is harmful to health. It can cause wind-deficiency due to rapid obesity, obstruct the vessels, weaken the sinews, bones and muscles. It brings on disease especially to those who suffer from incised wound. Those who take pork and drink wine ought not to sleep in the corn stalks. It is also said that white pigs with white trotters and cyan patterns are inedible. The kidney of pigs can help regulate the kidney qi, while excessive taking of it leads to kidney deficiency and long-time taking of it affects fertility.

猪心肝不可多食，无益，猪临宰惊入心，绝气归肝也。猪肝、鹌鹑同食，令人面生黑点。

Pig heart and liver, bearing no good for health, should not be taken

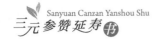

excessively as its fright and rage before slaughter enter into the heart and liver respectively. Taking pig liver and quail together leads to production of black spots on the face.

猪肉共羊肝和食之，令人心闷。不可与生胡荽同食，烂人脐。不可合龟鳖肉食之，害人。不可和葵及乌梅食之，气少；不可合鸡子同食，令人气消闷；食猪脂忌乌梅、生梅子，害人。

Taking pork and lamb liver together leads to chest distress. Pork may lead to fester of the navel if taken together with raw coriander, may impair health if taken together with turtle meat, may lead to insufficiency of qi if taken together with mallow and smoked plum, may lead to consumption of qi and distress if taken together with eggs. Pork fat is contraindicated with smoked plum and raw plum.

野猪青蹄者不可食。

Wild boar with cyan trotters is inedible.

江猪，多食体重。

Excessive taking of finless porpoise leads to the heaviness of the body.

豪猪不可多食，发风气，令人虚羸。凡煮猪肉用桑白皮、皂荚、高良姜、黄蜡块同煮，食不发风。脂油作灯，目暗。肝肺共鱼鲙或饴食之，作痈疽。共鲤子食，伤人神。八月勿食佳。脑子损阳，临房不能举。今食者以盐酒，是引贼也。曾不思皮尚可消而不觉其毒耶？头动风，其嘴尤毒，风人不宜。食者以竹叶烧烟撑口熏之，得口鼻涎出则无害。猪不姜食之，中年气血衰，面生黑黚。俞氏云："猪肉生姜同食，发疾风。"又云："发大风。"

Ericius should not be taken excessively as it may disturb wind and lead to deficiency and emaciation. Pork, if boiled together with Sangbai Pi〔桑白皮, White Mulberry Root-Bark, Cortex Mori〕, Zao Jia〔皂荚, Chinese Honey Locust, Gleditsia Sinensis〕, Gaoliang Jiang〔高良姜, Lesser Galangal Rhizome, Rhizoma Alpiniae Officinarum〕and yellow wax block, will not disturb wind. Lighting the lamp with the fat of pork blurs the vision. Taking the liver and lung of pigs together with minced fish or maltose causes carbuncle and deep-rooted ulcer. Taking it together with carps damages the spirit. It is better not to take pork in August. The brain of the pig affects potency, making men unable to have sexual activity. Presently, people take the pig brain together with salt and wine, which is similar with bringing danger upon oneself. How can they be unaware of the danger of it since it can even impair the skin? Taking the head of pig disturbs wind in the body and the mouth is especially harmful for those with wind syndrome. To make the pig mouth safe to take, one can burn bamboo and fumigate the pig mouth with smoke to let the saliva flow out. Taking pork with ginger leads to the declining of qi and blood and black moles on the face in middle age. Yu said, "Taking pork together with ginger leads to acute wind syndrome." He also said, "It can lead to severe wind syndrome."

羊肉性大热，时病愈，百日内不可食，食则复令骨蒸。和鲊食伤人心，

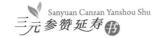
和生鱼酪食害人。生脂，宿有热者不可食。蹄甲中有珠子白者，名悬筋，发人癫。肝和猪肉及梅子、小豆食之伤人。心肝有窍，不可合乌梅、白梅食之，皆害人。山羊肉不可久食，及楮木炙食，及合鸡子食，令人腹生虫。大病人妊娠食肝，令子多厄。一切羊肝共生椒食之，破五脏，伤心，小儿亦忌之。肚子，病人共饭常食之，久成反胃，作噎病；共甜粥食之，多唾，吐清水。脑子，男子食之，损精，少子。欲食者，研细醋和之。猪脑亦然。不食佳。白羊黑头，食其脑作肠痈。饮酒后不得合羊、豕脑，大害人。心有孔者及一角者，皆杀人。

Mutton is greatly heat in property. It is not suitable for those just recovered from seasonal diseases within one hundred days. Otherwise, it may lead to hectic fever due to yin deficiency. Taking it together with salted fish damages the heart; taking it together with fresh fish and cheese brings harm to health. The mutton fat uncooked ought not to be taken by those with abiding heat diseases. The sheep with white beads in the trotters are called "Xuanjin", which may lead to epilepsy. Taking the sheep liver, pork, plums and red beans together impairs health. The sheep heart and liver are kinds of orifices, which are harmful to health and should not be taken together with smoked plum and white plum. Goat meat can not be taken for a long time as it may lead to parastic diseases if toasted by mulberry wood or taken together with eggs. Taking the sheep liver during pregnancy brings diseases to the infants. Taking the sheep liver together with pepper affects the five zang-organs and impairs the heart, which should be forbidden for children. Taking the sheep stomach as meals for a long time causes nausea and choking disorder; taking it together with sweet porridge brings on much saliva and acid water.

Taking the sheep brain affects the essence and fertility of men. It should be taken together with vinegar after grinding finely, so does the pig brain. It is better not to take it. Taking the brain of white sheep with black head causes carbuncle in the intestines. It is severely harmful to take the brain of sheep or pig after drinking wine. It is deadly to take the sheep with holes in the heart or with a single horn.

羖羊，青羝羊也。肉以水中柳木及白杨木，不得于铜器内煮。食之丈夫损阳，女子绝阴，暴下不止。髓及骨汁合食，烦热难退，动利。六月勿食，以益神气。

Ram is also called Qing Di Yang. Its meat can be boiled in water by burning willow or poplar, while it should not be boiled in the vessel made of copper. Otherwise, it may cause yang damage for men and endless vaginal bleeding due to yin damage for women. Taking its bone soup with marrow together leads to vexation, fever and diarrhea. It should not be taken in June to benefit the spirit and vitality.

青羊肝和小豆食之，目少明。

Taking the goral liver together with red beans blurs the vision.

羊不酱同食，久而生癞，发痼疾。

Mutton ought not to be taken together with sauce, otherwise it may lead to leprosy and bring on the chronic diseases.

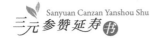
羊、猪血，人不可过，多食则鼻中毛出，昼夜可长五寸，渐粗圆如绳，痛不可忍，虽忍痛摘去，即复生。子益治奇疾，方用乳石、硒砂各一两为末，以饭丸如桐子大，空心临卧，水吞下十粒，自然退落。

Mutton and pork blood should not be taken excessively, otherwise it may lead to generation of 5 inch long hair as thick as rope inside the nose one day and night, which is unbearably painful and can regenerate again after plucking off. Zi Yi treated this odd disease with the formula composed of 1 Laing of Rushi〔乳石, Stalactite, Stalactitum〕and Selenium sand respectively. Grind them into powder and mix with rice to make into pills as big as seed of tung tree. Take 10 pills with water on empty stomach before sleep, the disease will be cured naturally.

牛盛热时卒死者，不食，作肠痈，下痢者必剧。丑月食之，伤神气。患牛脚蹄中拒筋，食之作肉刺。合马肉食，身痒；共猪肉食，生寸白。不可和黍米、白酒、桑柴火炙，并生栗食，生寸白虫。牛肉，患冷人不宜食。五脏各补人五脏。沙牛肉，常食发宿病。

It is not advised to take the beef if the cattle is hot to death suddenly, otherwise it may lead to intestinal carbuncle and aggravate dysentery. Taking it in December damages the spirit and vitality. Taking the sinews in the trotters may result in corn. Taking beef together with horse meat causes itch of the body; taking it together with pork causes the breeding of pin worms. Beef should not be taken together with broiled broomcorn millet and liquor by mulberry wood and raw chestnut, otherwise it may lead to production of pinworms. Beef is not suitable for people with cold syndromes to take. The five zang-organs of cow nourish the counterparts of people. Taking fried beef slice frequently may induce chronic diseases.

牛者，稼穑之资，不可屠杀。自死者，血脉已绝，骨髓已竭，不堪食。牛黄发病，黑牛尤不可食。牛乳汁及酪合生鱼食，成鱼瘕。花牛最毒，眼疾人吃双盲，用姜损齿。独肝牛肉食之杀人，牛食蛇者独肝。

Cows, as labor force in sowing and reaping, should not be slaughtered. Those naturally dead ones, exausted in blood, vessel and marrow, should not be taken as food. Yellow cows tend to induce disease and black ones are especially inedible. Milk and cheese, if taken together with raw fish, lead to abdominal mass. Cows with patterned skin are most toxic, leading to blindness for those with eye disorders and damage to teeth if taken together with ginger. It is deadly to take meat of cows with one liver, which is caused by eating snakes.

一切牛，盛热气时奇死者，总不堪食，生肠痈之疾。食牛之人，生遭恶鬼侵害，多染疫疠；死入地狱，受赦所不原之罪，戒杀编类。

Cows that are dead due to high temperature are inedible, otherwise they may lead to intestinal carbuncle. Those who take cows as food are likely to be invaded by devils, pestilence and epidemic disease when alive, to go to hell and suffer from unforgivable crimes like ahimsa after death.

台州摄参军陈昌梦入东岳，见廊下有罪数人，悉断割肢体，号叫极甚。陈问阴吏，曰："此数人以食牛肉，宰杀耕牛，受此报也。"既觉，

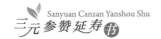

遂不食牛肉与鸡。台州起瘟疫，环城几无免者，陈颇忧之，梦神告曰："子不食牛肉，我当护卫。邪疫之气，各自回避，不必忧也。"其患遂息。好食牛肉，人寿禄皆减，百神皆散。戒食者，百神守护，妖邪鬼魅不敢侵犯。

Chen Chang, the temporary staff officer of Taizhou, once dreamed being in a place named Dongyue like the hell. There he saw several criminals in the corridor howling painfully for their dissected body and sliced limbs. Chen Chang asked the official in the nether world and he said, "They are suffering from the retribution because they killed farm cattles to take them as food." After this dream, Chen Chang never took beef and chicken anymore. Later, pestilence occurred in Taizhou and no one could survive it. Chen Chang was very anxious too and was told by a God in a dream as this, "You did not take any beef so I will protect you. Just keep away from the pestilence and there is no need to worry." Then the pestilence disappeared. Those who like to take beef can hardly occupy longevity and high rank, which are reduced by various Gods. Those who restrain from taking beef are protected safe by various Gods against Demons and ghosts.

马肉，自死者害人，甚者杀人，勿食。下痢人食者加剧。肉多着水浸洗，方煮得烂，去血始可煮炙，肥者亦然。不然毒不出，患疔肿。只可煮，余食难消，不可多食。妊不食。五月食之，伤神气。食肉而心烦闷者，饮清酒则解，浊酒则剧。不与陈食、米同食，卒得恶，十死九。姜同食，生气嗽，患痢，食心闷。血有毒，饮美酒解。白马玄蹄脑令人瘨；白马青蹄肉不可食；黑脊斑臂肉不可食；鞍下黑色彻肉里者，伤人五脏。马头骨作枕，令人不睡。食死马，勿食仓米，发百病。马汗气及毛，不可偶入食中，害人。汗不可近阴，先有疮，不得近马汗及肉汁、马气并毛等，必杀人。马筋肉，非十二月采者，宜火干。马心，下痢人不可食。马蹄夜目，五月以后，勿食之。肉不可与鹿膳同食。患疥人食之，令人身体痒。马肉不可热吃，伤人心。马、猪肉共食，成霍乱。

The meat of naturally dead horse is harmful to health and even can cause death, so it is forbidden to take. It can also aggravate dysentery. The horse meat should be fully soaked and washed to leach the blood before it can be fully cooked or roasted, so does the fat meat. Otherwise, the toxin of the meat cannot be removed and may lead to furuncle and swelling. It is better to cook horse meat with boiling method. The meat cooked by other methods are difficult to digest and inappropriate to take much. It is forbidden to take horse meat during pregnancy. It damages the spirit and vitality if taking it in May. The vexation and distress in the heart after taking horse meat can be relieved by drinking fine rice wine and it can be deteriorated by drinking unfiltered rice wine. Taking horse meat together with stale rice may lead to acute diseases and nine tenths of them may die. Taking horse meat and ginger together results in cough due to qi counter-flow, dysentery, and distress in the heart. Horse blood is toxic, which can be relieved by drinking wine. The brain of a white horse with black hooves can cause epilepsy. The meat of a white horse with blue hooves is inedible. The meat of horses with black spine and patterned limbs is inedible. The meat of horses with black meat under the saddle impairs the five zang-organs. The pillows made of horse skull may lead to insomnia. Do not take the meat of naturally dead

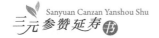
horse together with stale rice stored in the granary, otherwise it can induce various diseases. Horse sweat and hair should not be taken by mistake, which is harmful to health. Sweat should be kept away from things of yin property. So those who suffer from sores should not come near with horse sweat, horse meat juice, horse hair etc, which can lead to deadly diseases. Horse meat, if not obtained in December, is suitable to be dried by fire. Those suffering from dysentery should not take horse hearts. Do not take the horse hooves after May, otherwise it may lead to night blindness. Horse meat cannot be taken together with venison. Horse meat, if taken by those suffering from scabies, may lead to itching of the body. Do not take the horse meat when it is hot, otherwise it may cause damage to the heart. Do not take horse meat and pork together, otherwise it may result in cholera.

驴肉，病死者，不堪。骡、驴、马为其十二月胎，骡又不产妊，不可食。驴肉动风，脂肥尤甚，食肉慎不可饮酒，致疾杀人。尿稍毒，服不过二合。驴、猪肉合食，霍乱。醍醐酥酪有益无损，羊、牛、马酪食竟即食大酢，变血瀣，尿血。牛乳不可与酸物食，成坚积。驴乳冷，不堪酪。一切牛马乳及酪共生鱼食，成鱼瘕。乳酪煎鱼，主霍乱。

The meat of donkey dying of disease is inedible. Mule is the crossbreed of horse and donkey after the twelve-month pregnancy and it can not reproduce. So mule meat is inedible. Donkey meat, especially the fat meat, disturbs the internal wind in the body. Do not take donkey meat and drink wine at the same time, otherwise it may lead to fatal diseases. Donkey urine is slightly toxic if the amount is less than 2 He. Donkey meat and pork, if taken together, results in cholera. Curd cheese and finest cream are beneficial to health. Taking vinegar soon after cheese made from the milk of sheep, cows or horses leads to bleeding and hematuria. Milk should not be taken with food of sour taste at the same time, which may result in hard mass and accumulation in the body. Donkey milk is too cold in property to make cheese. The milk and cheese products of cattle or horses, if taken together with raw fish, lead to abdominal mass. Taking fish fried with cheese can cause cholera.

甲子日勿食一切兽肉，大吉。

On the day of Jiazi, the first day in the circle of Chinese calendar of heavenly stems and earthly branches, it is highly auspicious to take no animal meat.

《五行书》云：“白犬虎文，南斗君，畜之，可致万石也。”黑犬白耳犬，王犬也，畜之令家富贵；黑犬白前两足，宜子孙。白犬黄头，家大吉。黄犬白尾，代有衣冠；又白前两足，利人。人家养犬纯白者，主凶。

Wuxing Shu（《五行书》, *The Book of Five Elements*）says, "The white dog with tiger stripe is said to be the southern lord of constellation. Raise it as domestic animal and it can bring great fortune to the family." The black dog with white ears is said to be king dog. Raise it as domestic animal and it can bring wealth and rank to the family. The black dog with two white forefeet is beneficial for the offspring. The white dog with yellow head is

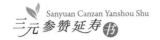
said to be propitious for the family. The yellow dog with white tail is said to indicate cultivation of scholar officials in subsequent generations. The yellow dog with two white forefeet is beneficial for people's health. The pure white dog is said to be ominous for the family.

犬黑色者，养之能辟伏尸。若斑青者，识盗贼则吠之。犬肉不熟食及多食，令人成瘕，患消渴病。

The black dog raised as domestic animal is said to be able to ward off zombie. The dog with black spots is said to be able to identify thieves and bark as warning. Taking uncooked dog meat or taking dog meat excessively can result in abdominal mass and consumptive thirst.

白犬合海鼬食，必生恶病。白犬自死舌不出，食之害人。不与蒜同食，损人。及悬蹄犬肉有毒，败人。犬瘦者，是病不可食。妊娠食犬，儿无声。九月禁食，以养神气。血，食肉而去血，不益人。狂犬，若鼻赤起与燥者，此欲狂，其肉不堪食。

White dog, if taken together with sea mink, can lead to malignant diseases. The white dog with its tongue unstuck out after death is deadly for people to take. Dog meat, if taken together with garlic, impairs health. Dewclaw of dog is toxic and unfavorable for health. The thin dog due to diseases is inedible. Taking dog meat during pregnancy may lead to dumbness of the baby. It is forbidden to take in September to help preserve the spirit and vitality. Taking dog meat with the blood removed is not beneficial to health. Mad dog whose nose is red and dry is to get rabies and its meat is not edible.

孙真人曰："春末夏初，犬多发狂，当戒，小弱持杖预防之。防而不免，莫出于灸。其法：只就咬处牙上灸，一日一次，灸一二三丸，在意灸至百二十日止。咬后便讨韭菜煮食之，日日食为佳。此病至重，世不以为意，不可不知也。"

Sun Zhenren（Sun Simiao）said, "In late spring and early summer, dogs tend to be restless, thus people should be on guard against this. It is better to frighten the dogs by holding a stick for the weak people. If bitten by a dog, moxibustion is a good treating method. Apply moxibustion on the wound once a day with three pills of moxa for 120 days. Take boiled leek immediately after being bitten by a dog and continue with it everyday. This disease, often received less attention, is very critical and need considerable recognition."

吃犬肉人，减克年寿（《戒杀编》）。人能戒牛、犬，寿命延长。

The longevity may be shortened and restricted for those taking dog meat as food [*Jie Sha Bian*（《戒杀编》, *Book on Abstention from Killing*）]. The longevity may be prolonged for those who are restrained from taking cow and dog meat as food.

《真武启圣录记》云："食犬折寿禄，作事大不利。"

Zhen Wu Qi Sheng Lu Ji（《真武启圣录记》, *The Record of the Great Emperor Zhenwu*）said: "Taking dog meat as food can cut short one's normal lifespan and reduce one's fortune, being unfavorable for all things."

鹿肉、獐肉为一，不属十二辰也。五月勿食之，伤神，豹文者，杀人。鹿茸不可以鼻嗅，有小虫入鼻为虫颡，药不及也。鹿肉痿人阴，不可近。

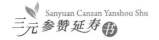
Venison and roe meat are of the same type and they are excluded of the twelve earthly branches. Do not take it in May, otherwise it may damage the spirit and those with the patterns of leopard is fatal to take. Do not smell pilose antler since small insects may enter the brain through nose, which is beyond the reach of medicinals. Keep off from venison for it can lead to impotency.

鹿肉, 多食令人弱房, 发脚气。麋不可合獭肉食之, 害人。不可合杂鸹肉食, 不可合生菜、虾米同食之, 害人。鹿角锉为屑, 白蜜五升淹之, 微火熬令小变, 曝干, 更携筛, 服之令人轻身, 益气, 强骨髓, 补绝阳。

Venison, if taken excessively, lead to impotence and beriberi. Elk meat should not be taken together with otter meat, otherwise it may impair health. It should not be taken together with francolin meat, lettuce and dried sea shrimp, otherwise it may be harmful to health. File the deer horn into powder, submerge it in 5 Sheng of white honey, decoct it with low fire until it becomes solid, dry it in the sun and take it after sieving. It can benefit health, replenish qi, reenforce the bone and marrow, and nourish the exhausted yang.

鹿一千年为苍鹿, 又百年化为白鹿, 又五百年化为玄鹿。玄鹿为脯, 食之寿二千岁。狸肉骨, 可治劳。

The deer that can live for 1,000 years long is called gray deer, that can live for another 100 years long is called white deer, that can live for another 500 years long is called black deer. The dried meat made from black deer can prolong one's longevity to 2000 years. The meat and bone of leopard cat can treat chronic fatigue syndrome.

白鹿肉和蒲白作羹，发恶疮。

Taking the soup made of white deer meat and cattail stalk causes severe sores.

壶居士云："饵药人食鹿肉，必不得效。以其食解毒之草，能散药力也。"

The lay Buddhist called Hu said, " Those taking venison during the process of meditation can not be treated effectively. The reason is that the deer often feed on herbs with detoxifying function, so their meat can reduce the medicinal efficacy. "

獐肉，八月至十一月食之，胜羊肉，余月动气。

Taking roe deer meat from August to November benefits people more that mutton. Whereas taking it in other months of the year disturbs qi of the body.

獐肉不可合虾及生菜、梅、李果实食，发痼疾。

Roe deer meat should not be taken together with shrimp, lettuce and plum, otherwise it may induce abiding ailment.

獐肉不可炙食，令人消渴。

Roe deer meat should not be toasted as food, otherwise it may lead to consumptive thirst.

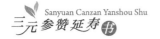

麂肉，多食动瘤疾。以其食蛇，所以毒。

Taking much muntjac meat brings on chronic illness because it is toxic for feeding on snakes often.

麋肉，不与野鸡及虾、生菜、梅、李果实同食，皆病人。

Elk meat should not be taken together with pheasants, shrimps, lettuce, plums and prugnas, which is harmful to health.

麋脂，不可近男子阴，令痿。肉不可与雉肉同食。

Elk fat should not be put near the male genitalia, otherwise it may lead to impotence. Elk meat should not be taken together with pheasant meat.

麋脂及梅、李子，若妊娠妇人食之，令子青盲，男子伤精。

Elk fat, if taken together with plum by pregnant woman, may lead to glaucoma; if taken by man, may lead to injury to the essence.

麋骨，可煮汁酿酒饮之，令人肥白，美颜色。

Elk bone, if decocted and made into wine, may make one strong and enjoy lustrous and improved complexion.

生麋肉共虾汁合食之，令人心痛。

Raw fawn meat, if taken together with shrimp juice, can lead to pain in the heart.

生麛肉共雉肉食之，作痼疾。

Raw fawn meat, if taken together with pheasant meat, can induce abiding ailment.

麋肉不可合鹄肉食之，成癥病。

River deer meat should not be taken together with swan meat, otherwise it may lead to abdominal mass.

麝肉共鹄肉食之，作癥病。

Musk deer meat, if taken together with swan meat, may lead to abdominal mass.

麝脐中香，治一切恶气、疰，百疾研服之，立瘥也。

Musk from the deer navel can be used to treat various pathogenic factors and chronic infectious diseases. Grind it into powder and take it, various diseases can be cured immediately.

象肉不可食，令人体重。

Elephant meat should not be taken as food, otherwise it may lead to heaviness of the body.

虎肉不可热食，坏人齿。虎肉正月忌食，以益寿。药箭死者，毒渍骨间，血犹能伤人，不可食。狸、豹同。

Tiger meat should not be taken hot, otherwise it may damage the teeth.

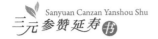

It is forbidden to take the meat of tiger during the first month of the lunar year to promote longevity. Do not take the tiger dying from poisoned arrow for its bones and blood having been poisoned through. The same is true of foxes and leopards.

人家畜猫一产止一子者，害其主人，急弃之乃免。又云：虽一产三四而皆雄或皆雌者，亦不可畜。

It is unfavorable for the owner if the domestic cat gives birth to only one kitten one time. Discard it and then the owner will be free from bad luck. It is also said that a litter of 3 or 4 male kittens or female kittens should not be raised as domestic animals.

兔肉，妊娠食，生子缺唇。兔产从口出，忌之宜。丹石人八月、十一月可食。多食损阳绝血脉，令人萎黄。痘疮，食之大毒，斑烂损人。二月勿食，养神气。共獭肉、肝食，成遁尸。鹅肉同食，血气不行。白鸡肝同食，面失血色，一年成疸。共姜、橘同食，心痛，成霍乱。

Eating rabbit meat during pregnancy leads to cleft lip of the baby. It is said that rabbit gives birth to baby through the mouth, so it is better not to take it during pregnancy. Those who take elixir can eat rabbit meat in August and November. Excessive taking of rabbit meat damages yang qi, blocks the blood vessels and leads to haggard and yellowish complexion. It is very toxic for those who suffer from smallpox to take and can cause fester and damage to their health. Do not take it in February to nourish the spirit and vitality better. Taking rabbit meat together with otter meat and liver causes acute disease with symptoms of abdominal distention and asthma. Taking it together with goose stagnates the circulation of qi and blood. Taking it together with the liver of white chicken results in pale complexion and jaundice a year later. Taking it together with ginger and orange causes heartache and cholera.

兔肉，深时则可食，令气全生。

Rabbit meat, if deep in color, is edible and can invigorates qi.

兔死而眼合者，食之害人。

It is harmful to take the rabbit with closed eyes when dead as food.

穿山甲，多食动旧风疾。

Taking an excessive amount of pangolin brings on chronic wind diseases.

豹肉，酸不可食，消人脂肉，令人瘦，损神情。

Leopard meat is sour in property and inedible. It may consume fat and flesh, lead to emaciation, damage the spirit and mentality.

獭肉，只治热，若冷气、虚胀，食之甚也。消阳，不益男子，宜少食。五脏及肉性寒，唯肝温，治传尸劳。

Otter meat can only be used to treat heat syndromes. For those who suffer from cold pathogenic factor or deficiency-type of distension, it may

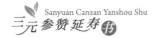
aggravate the diseases. It is not suitable for men to take much for its possible damage to the potency. Its internal zang-organs and meat are cold in property, but its liver is mild and can be used to treat infectious and severe diseases like tuberculosis.

熊肉，有痼疾者不可食，终身不愈。十月禁食。脂，不可作灯，烟气入目，失明。不可近阴，不起。

The bear meat is not suitable to take for people with chronic diseases, otherwise it may lead to incurability of those diseases. It is forbidden to take in October. Its fat cannot be used as the lamp-oil because the smoke it gives off may cause blindness. Keep it away from external genitalia for it can affect the potency.

麝肉共鹄肉食，作瘕。此物夏月食蛇，带其香，日久透关成异疾。不得近鼻，有白虫入脑，患虫颡。

Taking the meat of musk deer and swan together causes abdominal mass. Musk deer feeds on snakes during the summer months and smells of their odor, which can lead to unusual diseases with the odor invading inside. When bringing it near the nose, there may be pinworms inhaled through into the brain and causing parasitic diseases in the head.

猿猴，小儿近之伤志。

Ape and monkey may damage the mentality of children if approached.

猬肉可食，骨不得食，能瘦人，使人缩小。

The hedgehog meat is edible while its bone is inedible, which may lead to emaciation and contraction of figure.

肉汁在密器中气不泄者、禽畜肝青者及兽赤足者、有歧尾者、煮熟不敛水者、煮而不熟者、生而敛者、野兽自死北首伏地者、祭肉无故自动者、禽兽自死无伤处者、犬悬蹄沾漏肉中有星如米者、羊脯三月以后有虫如马尾者、米瓮中肉脯久藏者，皆杀人。

The following kinds of meat are deadly to take: the meat inside the enclosed container whose juice does not discharge out; the meat of livestock whose liver is blue and of beast whose hooves are red and tail is split; the meat that does not absorb water when cooked; the meat that can not be cooked fully; the raw meat that absorbs water; the meat of beast who dies naturally and falls on the ground facing the north; the sacrificial meat that moves by itself for no reason; the meat of birds and animals that die naturally with no wound on their bodies; the meat of dog whose feet is hanged over or whose meat is spotted with granules like rice; the mutton with worms like horsetail after being dried for three months and the dried meat stored in a rice urn for a long time.

脯暴不燥，火烧不动，入腹不消。自死，肝脏不可食。肉虽鲜，似有息气，损气伤脏。肉及肝落地不粘尘，不可食。诸心损心，诸血损血。一切脑、一切肝不可食，皆能害人。一切肉惟烂煮停冷食之，食毕漱口数过，齿不龋。食肉过度，还饮肉汁即消。禽畜五脏，三月三日勿食，

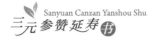

则吉。

The meat that is hard to dry after being exposed to the sun or to change after being burned with fire can not be digested. The liver of a naturally dead animal is inedible. The fresh meat with vitality damages qi and the internal organs. The meat and liver ought not to be taken if they are not contaminated with dust when dropped on the ground. Taking the hearts of animals as food damages the hearts of people and taking the blood of animals as food damages the blood of people. The brains and livers of all the animals are inedible and harmful to health. Meat should be boiled and cooked fully and kept cool before being taken. Then rinse the mouth several times to prevent dental caries. Excessive taking of meat can be relieved by taking the meat soup to help digest. It is auspicious to avoid taking the five zang-organs of the livestock on the third of March according to the lunar calendar.

鱼 类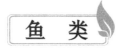

Fishes

鲩鱼及鳢鱼，有疮者不可食。

Grass carp and common carp are not suitable for people with sores to take.

鲤鱼，至阴之物也。其鳞三十六，阴极则阳复。所以《素问》曰："鱼，热中。"王叔和曰："热即生风，食之所以多发风热。"诸家所解皆不言。《日华子》云："鲤鱼，凉。"今不取，直取《素问》为正。万一风家使食鱼，则是贻祸无穷矣。

The carp, which has thirty-six scales, pertains to extreme yin in property. Extreme yin turns into yang. Thus *Su Wen*（《素问》, *Plain Questions*）says: "Fish brings on heat in the middle." Wang Shuhe said, "Heat can lead to wind syndrome, so taking fish can cause wind-heat syndrome." The above statements will not be discussed here. *Ri Hua Zi*（《日华子》, *Materia Medica of Ri Hua-Zi*）says: "Carp is cold in property." This view is not agreed here, while the statement from *Su Wen*（《素问》, *Plain*

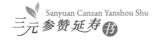

Questions）is taken as the right explanation. If a patient with wind syndrome takes fish by mistake, it may bring on endless damages to health.

鲤鱼多发风热，修理当去脊上两筋及黑血。沙石溪中者，毒多在脑，勿食其头。山上水中有鲤，不可食。五月五日，勿食鲤。

Carp may cause wind-heat syndrome if taken as food. The two tendons and black blood on the back should be removed before being taken. The toxin of carp living in streams with sand and gravel is mostly located in the brain, which should not be taken as food. Those carps living in the creek on the mountain are inedible. It is forbidden to take carp on May the fifth according to the lunar calendar.

天行病后不可食，再发痈疽。鲤鲊不可合小豆、藿食。食桂竟食鲤，成瘕。

People who have just recovered from epidemic should not take carp, otherwise it may cause carbuncle and abscess. Pickled carp is contraindicated with red beans or wrinkled giant hyssop. Taking carp right after fragrans causes conglomeration.

鱼及子不可合猪肝食，鲫鱼亦然。

Carp and its roe are forbidden to be taken together with the pig liver, and the same is true with crucian.

鳜鱼，背上有十二鬐骨，每月一骨，毒杀人，宜尽去之。

Mandarin fish has twelve hyena bones on its back, with each of them growing in each month of the year. The bone is toxic and deadly to take, thus it should be removed before eating.

苏州王顺食鳜，骨鲠几死。渔人张九取橄榄核末，流水调服而愈。人问其故，九曰："父老传橄榄木作棹，鱼触便浮，知鱼畏此木也。"

There was once a person called Wang Shun in Suzhou, who was almost choked to death by the bone of madarin fish. A fisherman called Zhang Jiu mixed the powder of olive nucleus with water and cured Wang Shun by it. When asked the reason, Zhang Jiu answered, " It is passed from forefathers that fish will die when running into the oar made of the olivine wood. Thus we got to know that fish is scared of the olivine wood."

白鱼，泥人心，疮疖人不可食，其发脓，灸疮不发。鲙食之，久食发病。

White fish may confuse the mind and it is not suitable for people with sores and furuncles to eat since it can cause pus. It has no effect on those with post-moxibustion sores. Taking it raw and sliced thinly for a long time causes diseases.

鲤鱼不可合犬肉食之。

Carp should not be taken together with dog meat.

六甲日，勿食鳞甲之肉。二月庚寅日，勿食鱼，大恶。

On the Days of Liujia, which refer to the six days when the heavenly

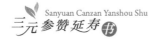

stem is Jia according to the Chinese calendar of heavenly stems and earthly branches to number the year, the month, the day and the hour, those animals with scale and shell should not be taken as food. On the day of Gengyin, which refers to the 27th day of Febrary, fish should not be taken as food, otherwise it may bring damgae to health.

鲫鱼，春不食其头，中有虫也。合猴、雉肉、猪肝食之，不宜。子合猪肉食不宜；和蒜少热；和姜、酱少冷；与麦门冬食，杀人；与芥菜同食，水肿。

The head of crucian should not be taken in spring since it has worms in it. It is not suitable to take together with monkey meat, pheasant meat or the liver of pigs. It is not suitable to take its roe with pork. Taking it together with garlic brings on slight heat syndrome; taking it together with ginger and sauce causes slight cold syndrome; it is deadly to take together with Maimendong ［麦门冬, Liriope, Radix Ophiopogonis］; it may lead to edema if taken together with leaf mustard.

青鱼及鲊，服术者忌之。合生葫、葵、蒜、麦、酱食不宜。

Those who are taking woody plants for the purpose of longevity are forbidden to take black carp or the pickled ones. It is not suitable to take it together with gourd, curled mallow, garlic, wheat or sauce.

黄鱼发气、发疮、动风，不可多食。合荞麦食，失音。

Yellow croaker can induce qi diseases and wind syndromes and cause sores, thus it should not be taken excessively. Taking it together with buckwheat leads to the loss of voice.

黄颡鱼不可合荆芥食，令人吐血，犯者以地浆解。

Pelteobagrus fulvidraco can not be taken together with Jingjie [荆芥, Fineleaf Schizonepeta, Herba Schizonepetae], which may cause hematemesis. This symptom can be relieved by slurry.

时鱼味美，稍发疳痼。

Shad is delicious but can cause chronic malnutrition.

魴鱼，患疳痢者禁之。

Gurnard is forbidden to take for people with chancroid dysentery.

鮎鱼勿多食，赤目赤须者杀人。合鹿肉及无腮者同。

Catfish should not be taken excessively. Those with red eyes and red palpus are deadly to take. It is also deadly to take it together with deer meat and the fish without gills.

鲻鱼久食，令人肥健。

Mullet can help people become strong and healthy if taken for a long time.

鲟鱼味美而发诸药毒，鲊虽世人所重，不益人。丹石人不可食，令

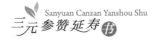
少气，发疮疥，动风气。小儿食之多成瘕及嗽。大人久食，卒心痛，合干笋食之瘫痪。

Sturgeon is delicious but it may induce the toxin of various medicinals. The pickled ones, though favored by people, are not beneficial to health. Those who take elixir should not take it as food because it may cause shortness of breath, sores and scabies, and disturb internal wind. The children who take it may suffer form conglomeration and cough. The adults who take it for a long time might suffer from acute heartache. Taking it together with dried bamboo shoots leads to paralysis.

鮸鮧鱼，腹中有子，最毒，不可食，令人下痢。

The puffer fish, if bearing eggs inside, is greatly toxic and inedible, leading to dysentery.

鲚鱼多食发疥。

The long-tailed anchovy，if taken excessively, may lead to scabies.

比目鱼，多食动气。

The flatfish, if taken excessively, disturbs qi inside the body.

鲈鱼多食令人发痃癖病，鲊尤良。肝不可食，中其毒，面皮剥落及疮肿。不可与乳酪同食。

The sea bass, if taken excessively, may lead to cord-like mass beside umbilicus. It is better to take it salted. Its liver should not be taken as food, otherwise its toxin may lead to epidermal desquamation, sore and swelling. It should not be taken together with cheese

鲫鱼不可同砂糖食，令人成疳虫。不可合乌鸡肉同食，令人发疸。

Crucian should not be taken together with granulated sugar, otherwise it may lead to infantile malnutrition and parastic worms. It should not be taken together with silkie chicken meat, otherwise it may lead to subcutaneous ulcer.

石首鱼，和莼菜作羹，开胃益气，只不堪鲜食。

Drumfish, if cooked together with water shield to make soup, can improve appetite and benefit qi. But it is not suitable to be taken fresh.

鳜鱼益气力，令人肥健，仙人隐，常食之。

Mandarin fish is beneficial for physical strength, making people strong and healthy. It is said the reclused immortals often take it as food.

章鱼冷而不泄。

Octopus is cold in property and may not cause diarrhea.

狗鱼暖而不补。

Pike is warm in property and has no tonifying function.

鲇鱼不可与牛肝合食，令人患风，多噎涎。又不可与野猪肉同食，令人吐泻。

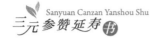

Catfish should not be taken together with calf liver, otherwise it may induce wind syndrome and choking due to saliva. It should not be taken together with wild boar meat either, otherwise it may lead to vomiting and diarrhea.

鳀鱼即鮀鱼也，不可合鹿肉食之，令人筋甲缩。

Anchovy, also called notopterid, should not be taken together with venison, otherwise it may lead to shrinking of tendons and nails.

河豚又名胡夷鱼，味珍。《经》云无毒，实有大毒，修治不如法，杀人。眼赤者害人，独行者不可食。食河豚罢，不可啜菊头。肝有大毒，中之立死。中其毒者，橄榄、芦根汁解之。

Globefish, also known as Huyi fish, is delicious. *Jing* (《神农本草经》, *Agriculture God's Canon of Materia Medica*) says it is non-toxic but actually it is extremely toxic. It can be fatal if not cleaned and processed well. Those with red eyes are harmful to health and those swimming alone in the water are inedible. After taking globefish, one should not sip tea of chrysanthemum head. Its liver is highly toxic and can lead to death immediately if taken. The juice of olive and reed rhizome can be used to detoxify its toxin.

鳜鱼，肝及子有毒，入口烂舌，入腹烂肠。

The liver and eggs of mandarin fish are toxic, leading to tongue fester if taken into the mouth, and intestine fester if taken into the stomach.

鱼即鼍也，老者多能变化为邪魅，又能吐气成雾。梁周兴嗣常食其肉，后患恶疮，切勿食之。

Sandfish, also called Yangtze alligator, can change into evil phantom and exhale to form mist when turning elderly. Zhou Xingsi of the Liang Dynasty often took it as food and consequently suffered from malignant sore later. So it should be forbidden to be taken as food.

鳅鱼，不可合白犬肉、血食之。

Loach should not be taken together with white dog meat and blood.

鳛鳝，不可合白犬肉、血食之。

Loach and eel ought not to be taken together with the meat and blood of white dogs.

鳝鱼，时病起，食之复，过则成霍乱。四月食之，害神气。腹下黄为黄鳝。又有白鳝，稍粗，二者皆动风气。妊娠食之，胎生疾。凡头中无腮，背有白点，并杀人。

Eel can be used to treat epidemic disease, but excessive taking of it can cause cholera. Taking eel in April is harmful to the spirit and vitality. The ones with yellow belly is called rice-field eel. There are also white eels, which are slightly thick. Both of the two kinds can disturb internal wind. If pregnant women take it, the fetus is prone to get diseases. The ones with no gills on the head and with white spots on the back are fatal to take.

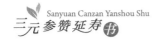

《茅亭客话》云："鳝、鳖不可杀，大者有毒，杀人。" 京师一郎官喜食鳝，一日过度，吐利大作，几殆，信不可多食也。

Mao Ting Ke Hua（《茅亭客话》, *Casual Chatting in Thatched Pavilion*）says: Eel and turtle should not be killed. The big ones are toxic and deadly to take as food. An assistant minister in the capital city was fond of eating eels. One day he ate too much and suffered from vomiting and diarrhea seriously, almost losing his life. Since then, he believed that eels should not be taken excessively.

鳝鱼肝生恶疮，勿以盐炙。食鳝，不可用桑柴煮之。

The liver of eel causes malignant sores if taken as food and it is not suitable to be roasted with salt. Eel should not be cooked with wood of mulberry.

鳝是赤圂，形类圣蛇，宜放，不可杀食。

Eel, resembling snake in shape, should be released instead of being killed and taken as food.

食鳝折人寿禄，作事无成。

Taking eel as food shortens one's lifespan and reduces one's salary, leading to failure of everything.

乌贼鱼久食，主无子。

Inkfish can cause infertility if taken for a long time.

乌鱼，水厌，焚修者忌之。

Mullet is the animal from water which is forbidden to take for those who practice Taoism, which is called "Taboo of Water".

鲎鱼，多食发嗽并疮癣。小者，谓之鬼鲎，害人。

Excessive taking of horseshoe crabs causes cough, sores and tinea. The small ones are called ghost horseshoe crabs and they are harmful to health.

鱼鲊中若有头发在内，误食杀人。

The salted fish with hair in it is fatal if taken by mistake.

黄鲿，食后食荆芥，杀人。

Taking Jingjie［荆芥, Fineleaf Schizonepeta, Herba Schizonepetae］ after yellow-head catfish is fatal.

凡一切鱼毒、鱼油点灯烟盲人眼，诸禽兽油亦然。无鳞恶荆芥，无腮发癫，全腮发痈。

The fish toxin and the lamp smoke emitted from the lighting of fish oil can cause blindness, which is also true of the oils of all kinds of birds and animals. The fish without scales is in mutual inhibition with Jingjie［荆芥, Fineleaf Schizonepeta, Herba Schizonepetae］. The fish without gills can cause epilepsy. The fish with gills can cause carbuncle.

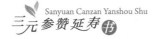

鱼目有睫、目自开合、二目不同、鱼连鳞者、无鳞者，皆杀人。

The fish that is born with eyelashes, with eyes opening and closing voluntarily, with different eyes, with scales the whole body or without any scale, is deadly for people to take.

腹下丹字鱼，煮不熟，食之成瘕。

The fish that is patterned with the Chinese character of Dan may lead to abdominal mass if taken uncooked.

石矾鱼勿食肠卵，就成霍乱吐泻。

Grouper's eggs should not be taken, otherwise it may lead to cholera, vomiting and diarrhea.

鱼无肠胆食之，三年，丈夫阴萎，女人绝产。

The fish without intestines or gallbladder, if taken for three years, may lead to impotence for men and infertility for women.

头有白色，如连珠至脊上者，杀人。白目、白背黑点、赤鳞、目合，并不可食。有角，食之发心惊。目赤者，作鲙成瘕，作鲊害人，共菜食作蛔、蛲虫。下痢者食鱼，加剧难治。

The fish with white spots on the head like a string of beads extending to the spine is fatal to take. The fish with white eyes, or black spots on white back, or red scales, or closed eyes, are inedible. The fish with horns on the head may cause palpitation. The fish with red eyes can cause abdominal mass if taken after being sliced thinly; they are harmful to health if salted; they can lead to parasitic diseases like roundworm or pinworm if taken together with vegetables. Those who are suffering from dysentery should not take fish because it may aggravate the condition.

一切鱼尾不益人，多有勾骨着人咽。

All the fishtails are not beneficial for health because they may contain hooked bones and cause injury to the throat.

鱼子共猪肝食，不化，成恶病。妊娠食干鱼，令子多疾。鱼汁肉不可合鸬鹚肉食。鱼鲙、瓜，忌同食。

Do not take roe and pig liver at the same time because it is hard to digest and tends to cause malignant diseases. Dried fish, if taken by pregnant women, may bring on the birth of a sickish baby. Fish soup should not be taken together with cormorant meat. Minced fish is forbidden to be taken with melons at the same time.

鳗鲡鱼，虽有毒而能治劳。

Anguilla can be used to treat consumptive diseases though it is toxic.

昔陈通判女，病劳将死，父母以船送之江中，漂泊孤洲，渔人见而怜之，与之鳗鲡羹，渐有生意。越月，渔人送还陈府，女病已脱然矣。

Once there was a state governor surnamed Chen. His daughter was dying of consumptive disease. The parents sent her to the river by boat and let her drifted on the water alone. A fisherman

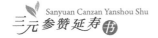

saw her and was very sympathetic, so he fed her with anguilla soup and gradually she came alive. A few months later, the fisherman sent her home recovered completely.

治蚊虫，以鳗鲡鱼干于室中烧之，蚊子即化为水矣。烧烟熏毡中蛀虫，置其骨于箱衣中，断白鱼蛀虫。

To kill mosquitoes, burn dried anguilla in the room and then the mosquitoes will be transformed into water. Moths in the felt can be driven out by the smoke given out by smouldering anguilla; whitefish moths can be removed by putting anguilla bone in the suitcase.

鳢鱼属北方癸化，不可杀，只宜放。能发疮，忌食。又能治脚气，风气食之效。

Snakehead fish, being originated from Gui（the last of the ten heavenly stems）of the northern part, should be set free instead of being killed. It should not be taken as food for it may lead to sores. It can treat beriberi and cure wind diseases.

南方溪涧中有鱼，生石上，号石斑鱼，作鲊甚美。至春有毒，不可食，云与蜥蜴交也。

There is a kind of fish living on the rock in the mountain stream of the southern part, which is named grouper and is delicious when pickled. It becomes toxic in spring and is forbidden to be taken as food. It is said that the grouper mates with lizard.

《真武启圣录》：大忌食鳖，系四足状，如神龟，只宜放，不宜杀，食折人寿禄，作事不利。

Zhen Wu Qi Sheng Lu （《真武启圣录》, *The Record of the Great Emperor Zhenwu*）says: It is a major taboo to take turtle as food. It is four-footed and looks like the supernatural tortoise. So it should be set free instead of being killed, otherwise it may shorten one's lifespan and reduce one's salary, exerting negative influence on everything.

鳖居水底，性甚冷。有劳气、癥瘕人，不宜食。肉主聚，甲主散。凡制鳖，当剉其甲同煮，熟则去其甲食之，庶几性稍平。目大者、赤足者、肉下有王字形者、三足者并能杀人。独目者、目白者害人。腹下有蛇纹者，是蛇，须看之。合鸡子、鸭猪肉、兔肉、芥子、酱，食之损人。

Turtle lives underwater and is extremely cold in property. It is not suitable for people with qi exhaustion due to over-strain or abdominal mass to take. Its meat has the function of gathering and its shell has the function of dispersing. When cooking turtle, file its shell and cook it with the meat together. When cooked, remove the shell and take the meat only. This can change its property from cold to mild. It is deadly to take such kind of turtles like those with big eyes, red feet, king-shaped patterns under the meat and three feet. Those with only one eye or white eyes are harmful. Those with snake-shaped patterns in the abdomen are snakes and they need to be distinguished with care. It is harmful to health to take turtle meat together with eggs, duck and pork meat, rabbit meat, mustard or sauce.

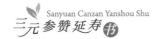

妊娠食之，令子短项。六甲日忌食龟、鳖及鳞甲，害人心神。薄荷煮鳖，曾杀人。合苋菜食，腹中生鳖。

If pregnant women take turtles, their babies may be short-necked. It is forbidden to take tortoises, turtles or their shells on the days of Liujia（the six days that are termed as Jia according to the calendar of the heavenly stem）because it may damage the heart and spirit. Turtles cooked with mint once led to death of people. Turtles, if taken together with amaranth, may lead to generation of turtle in the abdomen.

巢氏云：有主人共奴俱患鳖瘕，奴前死，剖腹得一白鳖仍活。有人乘白马来看，马尿落鳖上即缩头，寻以马尿灌之，化为水。其主曰：吾病将瘥矣。即服之，果瘥。

Chao Yuanfang said, "Once there was a master and his servant both suffering from abdominal mass due to turtle. The servant died firstly and then they dissected his belly and found a turtle alive. At this time, a man riding a white horse came to watch the scene. When the horse urine dropped on the turtle occasionally, it retracted its head. As a result, the turtle transformed into water when submerged in horse urine collected. The master said, "This is the method to treat my disease and I can be cured soon." So he took horse urine and was cured as expected.

龟黑者，常啖蛇不中食，其甲不可入药。十一月勿食龟鳖，能发水病。

The turtle that is black in color due to taking snake often is inedible and its shell ought not to be used as medicinal. Turtle should not be taken in November for it may cause edema.

龟肉共猪肉食害人；合酒并苽、白米、果子同食，令人生寒热；不可瓜食之；不可合苋菜食之。

Taking turtle meat and pork together is harmful for health. Taking it together with liquor, mushroom, polished rice and fruit leads to chills and fever. It should not be taken together with any kind of melon or edible amaranth.

六甲日勿食龟，害人心神。

Turtle meat should not be taken on the days of Liujia[①], otherwise it may damage one's mind.

蟹未被霜者，甚有毒，云食水莨，建音，人中之，不即疗，多死。背上有星点者、脚不全者、独螯者、独目者、两目相向者、足斑目赤者、腹下有毛、腹中有骨并杀人。中其毒，速以冬瓜汁、紫苏汤或大黄汁灌之。

The crab that has not experienced frost period is highly toxic. It is said that crab takes water ranunculus as food, which is read as Jian and is toxic. So people may die if invaded by this and untreated in time. It is deadly to take such kind of crabs like those with star-shaped spots on their back, incomplete feet, one claw only, one eye only, eyes opposite to each other, speckles on the feet, red eyes, hairs below the belly, bones inside the belly. Once poisoned, people should take white gourd juice, perilla soup or rhubarb juice as soon as possible.

---

① Days of Liujia: Six days termed as Jia of the heavenly stem according to the Chinese calendar of heavenly stems and earthly branches.

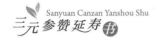
妊娠食之，令子横生。

If pregnant women take crabs, the fetus will be in a transverse position in the uterus at the time of birth.

蟹极动风，体有风疾、风气人，不可食之。

Crab tends to disturb wind in the body. So those with wind diseases should not take it.

至八月，蟹肠有真稻芒长寸许，向冬输与海神，未输芒，未可食。十二月勿食，以养神气。

In August, there are rice awns about an inch long in the crab's gut, which are to be sent to the sea god in the east as sacrifice. Before that, crabs cannot be eaten. Do not take crabs in December in order to nourish the spirit and qi.

食蟹即食红柿及荆芥，动风，缘黄下有风虫，去之不妨。与灰酒同食吐血。

It may disturb internal wind if taking red persimmon or Jingjie [荆芥, Fineleaf Schizonepeta, Herba Schizonepetae] immediately after crabs. The reason is that there is parasites under the crab cream which can lead to wind syndrome. Remove it and then it is safe to take. Taking crabs together with wine brewed with lime-water leads to hematemesis.

海边又有彭蜞拥出，似彭蝐而大，似蟹而小，不可食。

There is another kind of brackish-water crab on the beach in large number, which is bigger that Penghua（a kind of lodging crab）and smaller than crab. It is inedible.

蔡谟初渡江，不识而食之，几死。叹曰：读《尔雅》不熟，几为所误。

Cai Mo was nearly dead because he did not know this kind of crabs and took them as food when crossing the river for the first time. He sighed, "It was recorded and explained in *Er Ya*（《尔雅》, *Literary Expositor*）that this kind of crab is inedible. But I was not familiar with it and was almost died of it."

蛙骨，热食之，小便淋，甚苦。妊娠食之，令子寿夭。

The bone of frog is heat in property and may lead to painful stranguria. If pregnant women take it, their baby may die young.

蛙之小者，亦令多小便闭，脐下酸疼，有至死者，死者冷水擂车前草饮之。

The younger frogs may also cause stranguria and pain under the umbilicus. If the syndrome is deadly, mash Cheqiancao［车前草，Plantain Herb, Herba Plantaginis］and take it with cold water.

虾，发风动气及疮癣、冷积之疾。无须者，及腹中通黑煮而色白者，不可食。

Shrimp can induce wind syndrome, disturb qi, cause sores and tinea and diseases due to cold accumulation. Those without antennas, bearing black belly and turning white after being cooked are inedible.

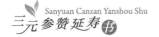

鲙虾、生虾不可合鸡肉，食之损人。鲊内有者，大毒。以热饭盛密器中作鲊，毒人至死。虾鲙共猪肉食之，常恶心，多唾，损颜色、精气。

Minced shrimps and raw shrimps, if taken together with chicken, are harmful to health. Salted fish with shrimps in it is greatly toxic. It is toxic to put people dead if taking the salted fish with shrimps and the hot rice in a closed container. Taking minced shrimps together with pork may lead to nausea, profuse saliva, poor complexion and impaired essence.

螺，大寒，疗热，醒酒，压丹石，不可常食。螺、蚌、菜共食之，心痛三日一发。蚌着甲之物，十二月勿食之。

Sea snail is extremely cold in property and is often used to treat heat syndrome, dispel the effect of alcohol and the side effect of elixir. It should not be taken frequently. Taking sea snail, clam and mussel together leads to heartache once in three days. It is not suitable to take clams in December for the possible pathogenic factors in their shells.

蚌冷，无毒。明目除烦，压丹石药毒。

Mussel is cold in property and nontoxic. It can be used to improve eyesight, remove vexation, treat toxicity of the elixir.

蚶子，每食后以饭压之，不尔令人口干。

Blood clam may lead to dryness of the mouth, which can be relieved by taking some rice after it.

蚶，益血色，利五脏，健脾，可火上暖之令沸，空腹中食十数个，以饭压之，大妙。

Blood clam can benefit blood and complexion, tonify the five zang-organs, and invigorate the spleen. Cook it on the fire until it is boiled, take a dozen on an empty stomach and then take some rice. It is of great good for health.

蛤蜊，服丹石人食之，腹中结痛。

Clam can lead to abdominal mass and pain for people who take elixir.

淡菜多食，烦闷、目暗，微利即止。

Mussel, if taken excessively, can lead to vexation, blurred vision and slight diarrhea.

蚬多食，发嗽并冷气，消肾。

Corbicula, if taken excessively, may cause cough, induce cold syndrome and impair the kidney.

马刀，京师谓之橦岸，发风痰，不可多食。

Horse mussel, also called Tong An in the capital, tends to induce phlegm due to wind pathogen and should not be taken excessively.

蛏与服丹石人相宜，天行病后不可食，切忌之。又云：主胸中烦闷，

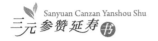

邪热相过，须在饭后食之佳。

Razor clam is suitable for people who take elixir and should be forbidden to take after the occurrence of epidemic diseases. It is also said that it is indicated for chest distress due to exuberance of pathogenic heat, so it is better to take it after meal.

虫 类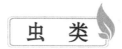

Insects

蜜，七月勿食生韭，发霍乱。蜜瓶不可造鲊，鲊瓶不可盛蜜，及蜜煎损神气。

Raw honey, if taken in July, can cause cholera. Do not make salted fish with the bottle that has been used to hold honey, and do not put honey in the bottle that has been used to hold salted fish. Fried honey damages spirit and qi.

白花蛇，用之去头尾，换酒浸三日，弃酒不用。火炙仍令去骨皮，此物甚毒，不可不防。

White-dappled snake should be submerged in wine for three days with its head and tail removed before being used. The wine should be changed daily and discarded finally. After that, bake it to remove its bone and skin. It is extremely toxic and need to be processed cautiously.

乌蛇，生商洛，今蕲黄有之，皆不三棱，色黑如漆，性善，不啮物，

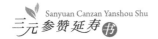

多在芦丛嗅花气，尾长能穿百钱者佳。市者伪以他蛇，烟熏货之，不可不察。脊高，世谓剑脊乌稍。

Garter snake grows in Shangluo and can also be found in Qihuang now. Its body is not triangular and its color is as black as paint. It is docile in temperament and does not prey for other animals. It often sniffs the smell of flowers in the reeds. The ones with long tails which can pass through a hundred copper coins are good in quality. In the market, it is replaced with other kind of snakes smoked black and then traded. This should be distinguished clearly. It is called "garter snake with sward-shaped spine" for its highly protruded spine.

商州有患大风，家人恶之，为起茅屋，山中有乌蛇，堕酒罂，病人不知而饮，遂瘥。《史记》有患者，食至胸即吐，作胃疾不愈。病者曰，素有大风，求蛇肉，风愈而此疾。盖蛇瘕，腹上有蛇形也。

Once there was a patient in Shangzhou who got leprosy and his family built a cottage for him in the mountain to prevent infection. Then a garter snake fell into the vessel of wine, and being unaware of it, the patient drank and got cured. *Shi Ji*（《史记》, *Historical Records*）says: There was once a patient who would vomit as soon as he took any food. It was treated as gastric disease but uncured for a long time. The patient said that he had previously suffered from leprosy and taken snake meat to treat it. Then his leprosy was cured but he suffered from the present disease again. This should be an abdominal mass due to snake because there was a snake-shaped lump in his abdomen.

蛇头不可以刀断，必回伤人，名蛇箭。

The head of snake, if cut off with knife, can turn back and bite people, which is called "snake arrow".

已年不宜杀蛇。见蛇莫打，损寿。凡见蛇交则有喜。

It is inappropriate to kill snakes in the year of Si（a method to mark the year according to the heavenly stem and earthly branches）. It shortens the lifespan to strike snakes. It brings good luck to come across snakes mating.

蛤蜊，其毒在眼，其功在尾，尾全为佳。

The toxicity of clam lies in its eyes and the efficacy lies in its tail. So the ones with complete tails are of good quality.

水蛭干者，冬月猪脂煎令黄，乃堪用，腹有子去之。此物极难死，火炙经年，得水犹活。

Sun-dried leeches can be used only after they are fried with pig fat to yellow in winter. Remove the spawns before being used. It is hard to kill leeches completely and it can come to life again in water even after being roasted on fire for a long time.

石蛭，头尖腹大，不可药用，误用令人目生烟不已，渐至枯损，不可不辨。

Shizhi, a kind of leech that lives among the rocks, is sharp in head and large in belly, which cannot be used as medicinal. It may lead to blurred vision and faded physique if used by mistake. So it should be distinguished

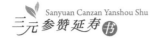

clearly before usage.

有吴少师得疾数月，肉瘦，食下咽，腹中如万虫钻刺且痒痛，皆以为劳。张蜕取黄土，温调服。下蚂蟥千余，皆困。云：去年出师饮涧水，似有物入口，吞入喉，自此得疾。夫虫入肝脾，势须滋生，食时则聚丹田间，吮哑精血，随则散处四肢，久则杀人，不可不甚也。

Once there was a patient named Shaoshi in Wu area who suffered from a disease for months and lost weight greatly. When he swallowed food, there was stabbing pain like the biting of thousands of insects and tickle torture in his abdomen, which was thought to be consumptive disease by all. A doctor named Zhang Tui asked him to drink the warm mixture of water and loess. Then more than a thousand leeches were discharged from his body, unable to move. Shaoshi said, "I drank the water in the mountain stream last year when marching army for battle. It seemed that something was taken into the body through the throat. Since then I got the disease." Therefore, when the leeches arrive in the liver and spleen, they grow and reproduce quickly. They gather in the elixir field to suck and sip essence and blood when hungry and scatter around the limbs when full, which may cause death for a long term. This must be known well.

蜈蚣，黄足者甚多，不堪用。
Centipede, mostly with yellow feet, can not be used as medicinal.

鸡杀过宿，收拾不密，此虫必集其中，不再煮而食之，其害非轻。
The chicken, if killed and kept for a night but not sealed well, must has centipedes gathering inside it. Taking such kind of chicken without cooking again can be severely harmful to health.

花蜘蛛丝最毒，能瘤，断牛尾，人有小遗，不幸而着阴，缠而后已，切宜慎之。曾有断其阴者。

The silk of the agelena is the most toxic type, which can even tie and break oxtail. When urinating, one should be cautious to prevent it from entangling the penis. It is said that someone's penis was broken off by its silk.

蚕沙煮酒，色清美，能疗疾病矣。

The wine boiled with silkworm excrement is clear and bright in color, which can be used to treat diseases.

蜘蛛灰色大腹，遗尿着人，作疮癣。

The urine of the spider in grey color with big belly can cause sores and tinea.

蚯蚓，暑月履湿，毒能中人。

The earthworm is toxic during the damp and hot summer and is harmful to health.

昔有中其毒者，腹大，夜闻蚯蚓鸣于身，以盐水浸之而愈。又张歆为蚓所咬，形如大风，眉须尽落，每蚓鸣于身，亦以此取效，仍当饮盐汤。

There was once a person who suffered from abdominal distention due to earthworm toxin. At night when he heard the sound of earthworms inside his body, he drank salty water to kill the

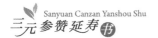

earthworms and was cured. There was another person called Zhang Xin who was once bitten by an earthworm and suffered from such symptoms like leprosy and loss of eyebrows and beard. When he heard the sound of earthworms inside his body, he used the same method of drinking salty water to treat it and was cured.

卷之四
Volume Four

明·钱塘胡文焕（德父）校

Collated by Hu Wenhuan from Qiantang County of Ming Dynasty

神仙救世却老还童真诀

The Pithy Formula of the Immortals Saving
the World and Renewing Youth

三元之道，所谓地元、人元，百二十岁之寿，得其术则得其寿矣。如迷途，一呼万里可彻然。天元六十者，固已失之东隅，能不收之桑榆者乎？归而求之，又将与天地始终，岂止六十而已哉？乔松彭祖，当敛在下风，或曰此道神仙所秘也。少火方炎，强勉而行真，可一蹴而造仁寿之域？奈之何！道不易知也，纵知之亦未易行也。人年八八，卦数已极，汞少铅虚，欲真元之复殂，渴而穿井，不亦晚乎？煮石为粥，曾不足喻其难，于是岂知道也哉？剥不穷则复不返也，阴不极则阳不生也，知是理可以制是数矣。《回真人内景诀》曰："天不崩地不裂，惟人有生死何也？"曰："人昼夜动作，施泄散失元气不满天寿，至六阳俱尽，即是全阴之人，易死也。"若遇明师指诀，信心苦求则虽一百二十岁，犹可还乾，譬如树老用嫩枝再接，方始得活。人老用真气还补，即返老还

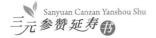
少。勤修一年，元气添得二两，便应复卦道。

Based on the Law of the Three Yuan, the Yuan of the earth and the Yuan of the human-beings amount to 120 years of lifespan, which can be attained by those following the methods of health cultivation. Pursuing the wrong path leads to the loss of lifespan, but it would be plainly clear once called back to the right path. The Yuan of the heaven enables people to possess another lifespan of 60 years. Since one has already lost in the East, how could he give up gaining in the West? Return to the right route and one will be endowed with the blessings of the heaven and earth and enjoy the lifespan of more than 60 years. Even Qiao Song and Peng Zu[①] would acknowledge the superiority of it. Or it is said that these methods are kept known only by immortals. Do not practice the health cultivation methods when one is too young just like the fire starting to flame. How could the longevity be realized overnight? The reason is that it is hard for one to perceive the methods and even harder to carry them out in practice. When people are in their sixties, they are at the end of their lifespan according to the Eight Diagrams. At this point, they are in severe lack of Gong (refers to the acquired qi) and Qian (refers to the original qi), so it is like digging a well while in thirsty if they want to restore the promordial qi. Isn't it too late to do so? It is very hard to describe the difficulty of these methods even with the metaphor of making porridge with stones. How could it be known clearly to people? According to the Eight Diagrams, the end of "Bo" gives rise to the birth of "Fu", the

① Qiao Song refers to two immortals in the ancient time, who are named Wang Ziqiao and Chi Songzi respectively. Peng Zu refers to a legendary figure of Taoism who lived for 800 years.

extreme of "yin" leads to the birth of "yang". Being informed of this rule enables people to hold their fate. *Hui Zhen Ren Nei Jing Jue*（《回真人内景诀》, *Key to Interior Scenery Practice of Hui Immortal*）says: The heaven doesn't collapse and the earth doesn't split. Why do human-beings undergo birth and death only? It says: People are in motion day or night, which leads to the loss of the vitality and shortness of the lifespan. When the essence of the six yang meridians is exhausted and only that of the yin meridians is left, people are inclined to die. If running across the guidance of a wise master and pleading with sincerity, one can still restore the vitality even at the age of 120 years old, just like grafting a tender branch onto an old tree to bring it back to life. One can rejuvenate with the help of genuine qi even at the old age. One year of diligent practice can increase the vitality by two Liang, which is in accordance with the diagram.

《书》曰：人者，物之灵也。寿本四万三千二百余日，元阳真气，本重三百八十四铢，内应乎乾。乾者，六阳具而未知动作施泄。迨十五至二十五，施泄不止，气亏四十八铢。存者，其应乎姤。加十岁焉，又亏四十八铢。存者，其应乎遁。加十岁焉，又亏四十八铢。存者，其应乎否。至此乃天地之中气。又不知所养，加五岁焉，其亏七十二铢。存者，其应乎观。加五岁焉，其亏九十六铢。存者，其应乎剥。剥之为卦，上九一阳爻而已。《仙书》曰："有一爻阳气者不死。"倘又不知所觉，则元气尽矣，其应乎坤。坤者，纯阴也，惟安谷而生，名曰苟寿。当此苟寿之时，而不为延寿之思，惑矣。天下无难事也。马自然怕老怕死，有六十四岁将谓休之叹，汲汲求道。遇刘海蟾传以长生之诀，返老还婴，

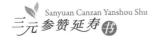
遂得寿于无穷。彼何人哉？晞之则时在一觉顷耳。苟能觉之体大易之，复日积月累，元气充畅，复而临，临而泰，泰而大壮，大壮而夬，真精纯粹，乾阳不难复矣。箕畴五福之一，微斯人吾谁与归？虽然此道天之宝也，有能觉之，天不负道，必将默佑于冥冥中，当遇至夫如刘海蟾者，以尽启其秘。滋补有药，导引有法，还元有图，则俱列于左。

The present book says: Human beings are the creatures with anima in the universe whose lifespan should be more than 43,200 days and original qi should weigh 384 Zhu, corresponding to the Qian Diagram interiorly. The Qian Diagram indicates the sufficiency of yang, which has not been released or consumed. During the period of 15 to 25 years old, people keep on consuming the original qi and a total amount of 48 Zhu is lost. Those left correspond to the Gou Diagram. During the next ten years, 48 Zhu is lost and those left correspond to the Dun Diagram. During the next ten years, 48 Zhu is lost and those left correspond to the Pi Diagram. So far, people mainly rely on the qi of heaven and earth to survive. During the next five years, 72 Zhu will be lost if they still neglect health cultivation and those left correspond to Guan Diagram. During the next five years, 96 Zhu will be lost and those left correspond to the Bo Diagram. At this time, only one yang trigram is left. *Xian Shu*（《仙书》, *Book of Immortals*）says: As long as there is one yang trigram left, people can still survive. The original qi will be exhausted if people continue to neglect health cultivation and those left correspond to the Kun Diagram, which is of pure yin property. In this stage, people can only depend on the cereal qi to survive, which is called the lifespan resigned to circumstances. So it is quite impenetrable if people still neglect health cultivation at this time. Nothing in the world is impossible. Ma Ziran, a Daoism immortal of the Song Dynasty, who was afraid of aging and dying, sighed at the age of 64 that it was time to the end of life, and endeavored to find ways to prolong life. Later, he met Liu Haichan, a Taoism master in the period of the Five Dynasties, who passed on the secret of longevity to him, and renewed his youth and enjoyed an infinite lifespan. What kind of person is that? He is just the kind that can be aware of this point. If people can realize the importance of the above laws and change their living patterns accordingly, the original qi will become sufficient and unobstructed again as time goes by. Then the Fu Diagram may transform to Lin Diagram, then to Tai Diagram, then to Dazhuang Diagram, then to Guai Diagram. At this point, the essential qi is pure and the Qian Diagram can be restored. Longevity ranks the first of the five blessings, which is among the nine categories of strategies created by Ji Zi to govern the world in the Shang Dynasty. Whom could I live together with if there were not such kinds of longevous people? Though this health cultivation method is treasured by heaven, people would not be let down if they could recognize and follow it just as being blessed somewhere. They may encounter immortals like Liu Haichan who could disclose the keys to longevity to them. Here listed are the medicines to nourish, methods to exercise and diagrams to restore the vitality.

滋补有药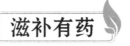

Medicines for Nourishment

孙真人曰："人年四十以后，美药当不离于身。"神仙曰："世事不能断绝，妙药不能频服，因兹致患，岁月之久，肉消骨弱。"彭祖曰："使人丁壮，房室不劳损，莫过麋角，妙药也。"

Sun Zhenren（Sun Simiao）said, "Nourishing medicinals are indispensable to people over 40s." The immortals said, "Earthly matters keep coming forth endlessly and good medicines cannot be taken frequently since it could induce diseases and cause emaciation and weakness of the body in the long run." Peng Zu said, "The antler of elk is an effective medicine to improve fertility and prevent sexual exhaustion."

麋角末七两，酒浸炙熟　　生附子一个，炮熟

Prepare 7 Liang of the powder of elk's antler, soak in liquor, bake until it is well done. Prepare 1 fresh Fuzi［附子，Prepared Common Monkshood Daughter Root, Radix Aconiti Lateralis Preparata］, process until it is well done.

上为末，合和，每服方寸匕，酒调，日三。

Grind the above ingredients into powder, mix and dissolve in wine, take one Fangcun Bi[①] of the decoction three times a day.

昔城都府有绿须美颜道士，酣酒楼歌曰：尾闾不禁沧海竭，九转丹砂都谩说。惟有班龙脑上珠，能补玉堂关下血。

In the past, there was a Taoist with green beard and decent appearance in city capital. Being satiated with liquor in the restaurant, he chanted, "If one suffers from the deficiency of kidney essence, none of the elixir could come into effect. Only the precious Bead on Banlong[②] head could supplement the kidney essence and nourish the blood by acting upon the Yutang acupoint."

乃奇方也，今名班龙珠丹。

The above mentioned chant is actually a magical prescription, which is called Banlongzhu Pill presently.

鹿角霜十两，为末　鹿角胶十两，酒浸数日，煮糊丸药　菟丝子十两，酒浸二宿，蒸焙　柏子仁十两，净，别研　熟地黄十两，汤洗，清酒浸二宿，蒸焙入药用

Prepare 10 Liang of Lujiaoshuang〔鹿角霜，Degelatined Deer-horn, Cornu Cervi Degelatinatum〕and grind into powder; prepare 10 Liang of Lujiaojiao〔鹿角胶，Deer-horn Glue, Colla Corni Cervi〕,

---

① Fangcun Bi: A measuring vessel in ancient time to take medicinal powder like a square-shaped spoon with the four sides one inch long.

② Banlong: refers to deer.

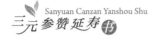

soak in liquor for several days, boil into paste and make into pellets; prepare 10 Liang of Tusizi〔菟丝子, Dodder Seed, Semen Cuscutae〕, soak in liquor for two nights, steam and bake it; prepare 10 Liang of Baiziren〔柏子仁, Chinese Arborvitae Kernel, Semen Platycladi〕, clean and grind separately; prepare 10 Liang of Shudihuang〔熟地黄, Prepared Rehmannia Root, Radix Rehmanniae Preparata〕, wash in boiled water, soak in liquor for two nights, steam and bake to make it ready for medical use.

上末，以胶酒三四升煮糊，杵一二千下，丸如梧桐子大，食前盐汤或酒吞下五六十丸。

Grind the above ingredients into powder, boil in three or four Sheng of Jiaojiu[①] to make it into paste, pestle it for one or two thousand times, then make into pills as big as the seeds of Chinese parasol tree. Take 50 or 60 pills with salty soup or wine before meals.

---

① Jiaojiu: a kind of medicated wine made of liquor, donkey-hide gelatin and salt.

导引有法

Guiding Exercise Methods for Health Preservation

夜半后生气时，或五更睡觉，或无事闲坐，腹空时宽衣解带，先微微呵出腹中浊气，一九止或五六止，定心闭目，叩齿三十六通，以集身中神气。然后以大拇指背拭目，大小九过，使无翳障，明目去风，亦补肾气。兼按鼻左右七过，令表里俱热，所谓灌溉中岳以润肺。次以两手摩令极热，闭口鼻气，然后摩面不以遍数，连发际，面有光。又摩耳根、耳轮不拘遍数，所谓修其城郭以补肾气，以防聋瞶。

At time when yang qi is rising after midnight, or when awake during three to five in the morning, or when sitting idle, or when on an empty stomach, one can undress the coat and untie the belt to get ready. First, breathe out the turbid qi from the abdomen slightly for nine times or thirty times. At this time, calm the mind, close the eyes, and click the teeth thirty-six times to concentrate the spirit. Then, wipe the inner and outer corners of the eyes nine times with the back of the thumb to prevent corneal opacity, dispel the wind pathogen and replenish the kidney qi. Press the left and right sides of the nose seven times to warm the exterior and interior part of the

nose, which is called "irrigating the Zhongyue area to moisten the lung" [1].
Then rub the hands till they are warm, hold the breath, and massage the face
for many times. Rub the hairline at the same time to luster the complexion.
Massage the ear root and auricle for many times, which is called "building
the city walls to replenish the kidney qi and prevent deafness" [2].

名真人起居之法：以舌柱上腭，上漱口中内外，津液满口作三咽下
之，如此三度九咽。《黄庭经》曰："漱咽灵液，体不干"是也。便兀
然放身心同太虚，身若委衣，万虑俱遣，久久行之，血气调畅，自然延
寿也。

Here is the living pattern of the immortals: Hold the tongue against
the upper jaw, rinse the mouth to generate saliva, swallow it in three times.
Repeat this for three rounds. That is the reason for *Huang Ting Jing*（《黄庭
经》, *Yellow Yard Canon*）to state like this: Swallowing saliva can moisten
and nourish the body. After doing this, it feels that the body is evacuated and
the mind reaches a state of great emptiness. It seems that one is as light and
carefree as getting rid of the shackles of clothes and worries. Keep practicing
like this for a long time and the blood and qi will be regulated, the lifespan
will be prolonged.

又两足心涌泉二穴，能以一手举足，一手摩擦之百二十数，疏风去

---

[1] irrigating the Zhongyue area to moisten the lung: This is a term of health preservation in TCM,
meaning to massage the two sides of the nose to benefit the lung.

[2] building the city walls to replenish the kidney qi and prevent deafness: This is a term of guiding
exercise in TCM, meaning to massage the ear to replenish the kidney.

湿健脚力。

One can also lift one foot with one hand and massage the Yongquan acupoint（KI 1）of the sole for 120 times with the other hand, which can dispel the wind pathogen, remove dampness and strengthen the feet.

欧阳文忠公用此有大验。

Ouyang Xiu, a statesman and writer of Northern Song Dynasty, used this method and acknowledged that it had miraculous effects.

神枕法：昔太山下有老翁者，失其名姓，汉武帝东巡见老翁锄于道傍，背上有白光高数尺。帝怪而问之有道术否？老翁对曰："臣昔年八十五时，衰老垂死，头白齿落。有道士者教臣服枣，饮水绝谷，并作神枕法，中有三十二物，其三十二物中，二十四物药以当二十四气，其八 物毒以应八风。臣行之转少，白发返黑，堕齿复生，日行三百里。臣今年一百八十岁矣，弃世入山，顾恋子孙，复还食谷，又已二十余年，犹得神枕之力，往不复老。"武帝视老翁颜状当如五十许人，验问其邻，皆云信。帝乃从受其方作枕，而不能随其绝谷饮水也。方用五月五日、七月七日取山林柏以为枕，长一尺二寸，高四寸，空中容一斗二升。以柏心赤者为盖，厚二分，盖致之令密，又当使可开用也。又钻盖上为三行，每行四十孔，凡一百二十孔，令容粟米大。其用药：芎䓖、当归、白芷、辛夷、杜衡、白术、藁本、木兰、蜀椒、官桂、干姜、防风、人参、桔梗、白薇、荆实、飞廉、柏实、白术、秦椒、麋芜、肉苁蓉、薏苡仁、款冬花，凡二十四物以应二十四气；加毒者八物以应八风：乌头、附子、藜芦、皂荚、甘草、矾石、半夏、细辛。

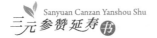

Divine pillow method: Once upon a time, there lived an elderly man near the Mountain Tai whose name was unknown. Emperor Wu of the Han Dynasty, on his eastern tour, was surprised to see a white light as high as several Chi above this elderly man who was laboring with a hoe beside the road then. So Emperor Wu asked him whether he was capable of theurgy or not. The elderly man replied, "I became old and feeble with white hair and loss of teeth when I was 85 years old. Then a Taoist taught me the method to keep fasting, during which I only took jujube and drank water, and the divine pillow method, which was to put 32 kinds of substances in the pillow. Among the 32 kinds of substances, 24 kinds are medicinal substances corresponding to the Twenty-Four Solar Terms, 8 kinds are toxic substances dealing with the 8 wind pathogens. Helped with the two methods, I became younger with white hair turning black and lost teeth reborn and was capable of walking for 300 Li (150 kilometres) within a day. I am 180 years old this year and living near the mountain away from the secular society. To care for the children and grandchildren, I gave up fasting and took meals as before. Twenty years have passed and I got unchanged thanks to the benefit of the divine pillow method." Emperor Wu observed the elderly man carefully, who looked like a man in his fifties, and verified from his neighbors who confirmed the authenticity of his words. So Emperor Wu, though unable to keep fasting, followed the method to make a divine pillow as this: Cut cypress from the mountain forest on May 5th or July 7th, and make a pillow out of it with the length of 12 Cun, the width of 4 Cun and the capacity of 12 Sheng. Make a 2-Fen-thick lid for the pillow with cypress whose central part is red. The lid, if covered, can enclose the pillow tightly and, if taken away, open the pillow. Drill 3 lines of holes as big as maize on the lid with 40 holes in each line, amounting to 120 in all. The medicinal herbs contained in the pillow include: Xiong Qiong［芎 劳，Sichuan Lovage Rhizome, Rhizoma Ligustici Chuanxiong］, Danggui［当 归，Chinese Angelica, Radix Angelicae Sinensis］, Baizhi［白芷，Dahurian Angelica Root, Radix Angelicae Dahuricae］, Xinyi［辛夷，Biond Magnolia Flower, Flos Magnoliae］, Duheng［杜衡，Forbes Wildginger, Asarum Forbesii Maxim］, Baizhu［白术，White Atractylodes Rhizome, Rhizoma Atractylodis Macrocephalae］, Gaoben［藁本，Chinese Lovage, Rhizoma Ligustici］, Mulan［木兰，Magnolia, Magnolia Liliiflora Desr］, Shujiao ［蜀椒，Pricklyash Peel, Pericarpium Zanthoxyli］, Guangui［官桂，Cassia Bark, Cortex Cinnamomi］, Ganjiang［干姜，Dried Ginger, Rhizoma Zingiberis］, Fangfeng［防风，Divaricate Saposhnikovia Root, Radix Saposhnikoviae］, Renshen［人参，Ginseng, Radix Ginseng］, Jiegeng［桔梗，Platycodon Root, Radix Platycodonis］, Baiwei［白薇，Blackend Swallowwort Root, Radix Cynanchi Atrati］, Jingshi［荆实，Hempleaf Negundo Chastetree Leaf, Folium Viticis Negundo］, Feilian［飞廉，Carduus armenus, Carduus nutans L.］, Baishi ［柏实，Chinese Arborvitae Kernel, Semen Platycladi］, Baizhu［白术， White Atractylodes Rhizome, Rhizoma Atractylodis Macrocephalae］, Qinjiao［秦椒，Pricklyash Peel, Pericarpium Zanthoxyli］, Miwu［麋芜， Sichuan Lovage Rhizome, Rhizoma Ligustici Chuanxiong］, Roucongrong ［肉苁蓉，Desertliving Cistanche, Herba Cistanches］, Yiyiren［薏苡仁， Coix Seed, Semen Coicis］, and Kuandonghua［款冬花，Common Coltsfoot Flower, Flos Farfarae］. The 24 kinds of medicinal herbs above correspond

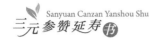
to the Twenty-Four Solar Terms. There are still 8 toxic medicinal substances added to confront the 8 kinds of wind pathogens: Wutou〔乌头, Aconite Main Root, Aconitum Carmichaelii Debeaux〕, Fuzi〔附子, Prepared Common Monkshood Daughter Root, Radix Aconiti Lateralis Preparata〕, Lilu〔藜芦, Hellebore, Veratrum Nigrum L.〕, Zaojia〔皂荚, Chinese Honey Locust, Gleditsia Sinensis Lam〕, Gancao〔甘草, Liquorice Root, Radix Glycyrrhizae〕, Fanshi〔矾石, Alum, Alumen〕, Banxia〔半夏, Pinellia Tuber, Rhizoma Pinelliae〕, and Xixin〔细辛, Manchurian Wildginger, Herba Asari〕.

上三十二物各一两，俱㕮咀，以此药上安之满枕中，用布囊以衣，枕百日面有光泽。一年体中所疾及有风疾一一皆愈，满身尽香。四年白发变黑，齿落更生，耳目聪明，神方有验，秘不传其非人也。藁本是老川芎母也，武帝以问东方朔，答曰："昔女廉以此方传玉青，玉青以传广成子，广成子以传黄帝。近者，谷城道士淳于公枕此药枕耳，百余岁而头发不白。夫病之来皆从阳脉起，今枕药枕，风邪不得侵入矣。又当以布囊衣枕，复以帏囊重包之，须欲卧枕时乃脱去之耳。"帝大喜，诏赐老翁匹帛，老翁不受。曰："陛下好善，故进之耳。"

Take 1 Liang of the above mentioned 32 kinds of medicinal herbs respectively, break them into small pieces, wrap them with cloth bag and put it into the pillow. Using the pillow for 100 days, one will enjoy improved complexion, get the abiding ailment of the year and the disease caused by wind pathogen cured, and bear fragrant scent. Using the pillow for 4 years, one will get white hair turned black, lost teeth reborn, hearing and eyesight improved as sharp as before. The efficacy of this formula has been proved and it was kept as a secret to avoid being misused by wrong people. Here, Gaoben〔藁本,Chinese Lovage, Rhizoma Ligustici〕 refers to the Szechuan Lovage Rhizome produced in Sichuan province. Emperor Wu once asked Dongfang Shuo about this pillow, who was a humorous litterateur and attendant officer then. Dongfang Shuo replied, "In ancient times, this formula was passed from Nvlian[1] to Yuqing, then from Yuqing to Guang Chengzi, then from Guang Chengzi to Huangdi. In recent times, Chun Yuyi, a Taoist of Gu city in Han Dynasty, used this medical pillow and kept his hair black when he was more than 100 years old. It is because the diseases are mostly caused by pathogenic factors invading yang meridians and the medical pillow can prevent wind pathogens from attacking inside. The medical pillow should be wrapped with cloth bag and then put in curtain bag when unused. The two bags should be taken off when one is to rest on the pillow." Emperor Wu was very pleased and ordered to grant silks to the elderly man as reward. The elderly man refused and said, "It is because of the benevolence of Your Majesty that I would like to present the formula."

---

① Nvlian, Yuqing, Guang Chengzi: They are medical practicers of Daoism in ancient times.

神仙警世

Cautionary Remarks from Immortals

　　黄帝问气之盛衰，岐伯对曰："人生十岁，五脏始定，血气通，真气在下，好走；二十岁血气始盛，肌肉方长，好移；三十岁五脏大定，肌肉坚固，血气盛满，好步；四十岁脏腑十二筋脉皆大盛以平定，腠理始疏，荣华颓落，发颇斑白，平盛不摇，好坐；五十岁肝气始衰，肝叶始薄，胆汁始灭，目始不明；六十岁心气始衰，善忧悲，血气懈惰，好卧；七十岁脾气虚，皮肤枯；八十岁肺气衰，魄离，故言善误；九十岁肾气焦，四脏经脉虚；百岁五脏皆虚，神气乃去，形骸独居。"

When Huangdi asked the exuberance and decline of qi during the course of a person's life, Qibo said, "When a person is 10 years old, the development of the five zang-organs is completed, the blood and qi in his body flow thoroughly through the body. At this period of physiological development, qi mainly circulates in the lower part of the body. That is why he likes to run. When he is 20 years old, blood and qi in his body begin to become exuberant and the muscles are fully developed. That is why he likes to walk quickly. When he is 30 years old, the five zang-organs are fully developed, the muscles are strong and hard and the blood vessels are full. That is why he likes to walk with firm steps. When he is 40 years old, the five zang-organs, the six fu-organs and the twelve channels are all perfectly developed and maintain stable, the muscular interstice begins to become flabby, the luster over the face begins to recede, the hair begins to turn white, the essence and qi have reached the peak and begin to decline. That is why he likes to sit down. When he is 50 years old, the liver-qi begins to decline, the liver lobe begins to become thin, the bile begins to reduce and the eyes begin to become blurred. When he is 60 years old, the heart-qi starts to decline, the emotional changes of anxiety, grief and sorrow begin to perplex him, blood and qi become weak. That is why he likes to lie on bed. When he is 70 years old, the spleen-qi becomes deficient and the skin becomes withered. When he is 80 years old, the lung-qi has declined and the corporeal soul has left the body. That is why he often makes mistakes in speaking. When he is 90 years old, the kidney-qi is exhausted and the channels of the four zang-organs are extremely deficient. When he is 100 years old, the five zang-organs are deficient, and the spirit and qi are exhausted. Though the body still remains, the life no longer exists."

《经》曰："人年四十阴气倍；五十肝气衰；六十筋不能动，精气少，须当自慎自戒，少知调和摄养，宁不为养生之本；七十以上，宜取性自养，不可劳心苦形冒寒暑。若能顺四时运气之和，自然康健延年，苟求贪得，尚如壮岁，不知其可如矣。"

Jing（《经》, *Medical Classic*）says: When one is in his 40s, his yin qi doubles. When one is in his 50s, his liver qi declines. When one is in his

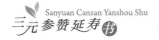

60s, his tendons are unable to move flexibly and his essential qi fades, so one should be cautious and restrain from bad habits, know the ways to harmonize and preserve health, and solidify the foundation of health. When one is in his 70s, he'd better preserve health in accordance with his own temperament instead of overworking the brain and body and exposing himself in cold and heat. If one can conform to the change of four seasons and the five kinds of movements and six kinds of climates, he is sure to remain healthy and longevous. If one still remains greedy and worries about personal gains and losses as he is in the prime period, he will feel powerless due to the age factor.

《壮神真经》曰：养生以不损为延年之术。不损以有补为卫生之经，处安虑危防未萌也，不以小恶为无害而不去，不以小善为无益而不为。虽少年致损，气弱体枯，及晚景得悟，防患补益，气血有余而神自足矣，则自然长生延寿也。

Zhuang Shen Zhen Jing（《壮神真经》, *Good Experience in Strengthening the Spirit*）says: Health preservation regards the method to avoid impairment as the art of extending life, which further takes nourishing as the way to maintain health. This view is to prevent diseases beforehand just like preparing for danger in times of peace. It is suggested to eliminate trifling evil though its damage is not so severe, to do tiny good deed though its benefit is not so great. Those who got infirmness in qi and physique due to certain kind of impairment during young ages can still enjoy a long and healthy lifespan if they can realize the importance of prevention and tonification and take measures to replenish qi and blood and to maintain mental health.

阴德延寿论

On Life Extension by Hidden Virtue

一念所觉，因所以得三元之寿，考一德之修，又所以培三元之寿脉甚矣。念之不可以不觉，而德之不可以不修也。老子曰："我命在我，不在天。"紫阳真人曰："大药修之有易难也，须由我也。由天若非积行施阴德，动有群魔作障，缘是可以自信矣。"道人郭太史，精于谈天者也，应天有书，后之星翁推步，必来取法。曰："五行四柱曰星辰运限如是，而富贵寿考如是，贫贱疾苦如是，而凶恶夭折若镜烛影，若契合符，世之人似不能逃其数者及其究也。合于书者固多，其不合者亦不少，是何欤？岂人生宇宙间，或囿于数，或不囿于数欤？盖尝考之。其推玄究微，既条列于前，至其后则曰："阴功不延其寿，吉人依旧无凶。"又曰："随时应物行方便，纵犯凶星亦不危。"是必有见矣。不然，寿夭休论命，修行本在人。

The longevity of three Yuan can be attained by awakening of the thought, and the longevous pulse of three Yuan can be developed by cultivating morality. The thought must be awakened and the morality must be cultivated. Lao Zi said, "I can not leave my whole life to fate." Ziyang

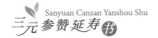
Sage said, "It is up to me to select the simple or hard medicinal method to maintain health. There would exist hindrance inflicted by devils on the way to health if it were not for the accumulation and performance of hidden virtue. Thus one should be self-confident in this aspect." There was once a Taoist named Guo, working as a court historian, who was good at the research of natural laws and had obtained relevant books bestowed by heaven. Whenever his friend named Zhi Xing calculated astronomical phenomena and calendar, he was bound to come to him for consultation. He said, "It is true for the fortune-telling method to be based on the five elements and four columns (namely the year, the month, the day and the hour of one's birth), and also the motion of stars. Someone enjoys wealth, rank and long lifespan; someone suffers from poverty, destitution and hardships; someone meets with vicious things and dies young. So life is something like the candle shadow reflected in the mirror and magic figure carved and drawn by Taoist priests. It is hard for people to change their predestined fate. When explored further, some cases are in accordance with what is stated in the book while some are not. What is the reason then? Is it because some people are constrained by fate while some others are not? I have attempted to carry out some textual researches to ratiocinate the mysterious rules and probe into the delicate facts." In the former part of the book, the results are classified and listed; in the latter part of the book, it says: Hidden virtue can hardly prolong lifespan and good people meet with no bad luck. It also says: Keep oneself in correspondence with the universe and make things convenient for others. Then one may be protected from danger even in terrible situations. There

must be some sound judgement in this sentence. Otherwise, the longevity and immature death would not be related with destiny and people should cultivate themselves by practice for a better life.

孙思邈曰："何以有此言欤？"

Sun Simiao said, "Why is it said like this?"

太极真人徐来勒尝遇南斗寿星，问寿夭吉凶之事。星君曰："天道福善祸淫，神明赏善罚恶逆。人能刻意为善，静与道合，动与福会，如此则我命在我，不为司杀所执，不求寿而自寿，不求生而自生。苟或堕纲纪，违天地，肆愚悖，侮神明，背仁慈，亏忠孝，明则刑纲理之，幽则鬼神诛之，是不知所积，冥冥中夺其算而夭其寿者矣。广行阴德如于公治狱，子为丞相。"徐卿积善，衮衮公侯，在所不论。昔比丘得六神通，与一沙弥同处林野间。比丘知沙弥七日当死，因曰"父母思汝可暂归，八日复来。"沙弥八日果来，比丘怪之入三昧。察其事，乃沙弥于归路中脱褧裳壅水，令不得入蚁穴，得延寿一纪。孙叔敖儿时见两头蛇，恐他人又见，杀而埋之。母曰："吾闻有阴德者，天报之福，汝不死也。"后为楚令尹。

Xu Laile, the master of Tai Ji, once met the God of Longevity in the southern constellation and inquired him about the matters related with longevity and divination. The God of Longevity said, " It is the natural law to bless the kind and curse the evil and it is the wisdom of God to award the good and punish the vicious. If people can do good deeds intentionally, correspond with the natural law when in tranquil and conform to happiness

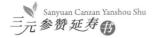

when in motion, then their fate can be governed by themselves instead of the slayer. They may enjoy longevity and vitality without painstaking striving. If people break the social order and rules, violate the natural laws, unbridle the ignorance and revolt, humiliate the Gods, abandon benevolence, lack loyalty and filial piety, then they would be rectified by criminal law and discipline alive and be punished by ghosts and Gods after death. The reason is that they have no idea that the accumulated wrongdoings may take their fortune and longevity away somewhere unseen. There are some examples about getting rewarded by cultivating hidden virtue extensively, such as official Yu of the Han dynasty, who was impartial in dealing with prison suits and had his son benefited to be the prime minister." And minister Xu, who insisted on doing good deeds, had his sons benefited to be dukes successfully. In the past, a Buddhist monk was endowed with six supernatural powers and lived together with an acolyte in the wild land. Knowing the acolyte bound to die in seven days by fate, the Buddhist monk said to him, "You can go home to visit your parents for they miss you very much. You may come back in 8 days. " Then the acolyte really came back after 8 days and the Buddhist monk was surprised and tried to check it in samadhi. It was found out that the acolyte took off his cassock to block water in case the ant cave may be drowned on his way home. For this reason, the acolyte got his lifespan prolonged with another 12 years. Sun Shuao once encountered a two-headed snake during his childhood and, to prevent it from hurting other people, killed and buried it. His mother said, " I heard that those with hidden virtue could be blessed with good luck, so you would enjoy a long lifespan." Sun Shuao was appointed as the prime minister of Chu State later.

窦禹钧夜梦祖父谓曰："汝年过无子，又寿不永，当早修阴德。"
禹钧自是勤修阴德，行之罔倦。后又梦其祖父与曰："天以汝阴德，故
延寿三纪，赐五子，荣显后，居洞天之位。"范仲淹为之记。由是观之，
三元寿考，固得于一念之觉，三元寿脉，又在于一德之修也。或曰：阴
德曷从而修之？曰：凡可修者，不以富贵贫贱拘，亦不在勉强其所为，
但于水火、盗贼、饥寒、疾苦、刑狱逼迫、逆旅狼狈、险阴艰难，至于
飞、潜、动、植，于力到处种种，多行方便，则阴德无限量，而受报如
之矣。善乎！《西山之记》曰：至人得传真法，虽云修养所至，是亦阴
德之报也。此予所以于参赞书后，复作论曰：阴德延寿。

Dou Yujun, a famous minister and book collector in the Five Dynasties
Period, once met his grandfather in dream who said, " You are destined to
bear no children and a short lifespan. To change this, you need to do good
deeds and accumulate merits as early as possible." From then, Dou Yujun
did many good deeds tirelessly to help other people. Later, his grandfather
said to him again in dream, "Regarding all the good deeds you have done,
you are blessed with additional 36 years of lifespan, a heavenly abode after
death, and five sons who will enjoy rank and honour." This story was
recorded by Fan Zhongyan, a famous statesman and writer of the Song
Dynasty. Therefore, the longevity of the three Yuan can be achieved not only
by the recognition of its importance in thought, but also in the practice of
cultivating hidden virtue. Someone may ask: How to cultivate hidden virtue?
This is the reply: It should not be managed reluctantly and be constrained

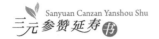

by wealth or poverty. It is believed to be infinite virtue and highly rewarding for people to provide various aid and convenience for those suffering from water and fire disasters, robbers, hunger and cold, disease and hardships, imprisonment and torture, awkward journey, dangers and troubles, and for the flying birds, swimming fishes, animals and plants. *Xi Shan Zhi Ji*（《西山之记》, *The Story of Western Hills*）says: The reason for the lofty person to get true Dhamma lies not only in the practice and exercise, but also in the the merits accumulated. This also explains why the chapter "On Life Extension by Hidden Virtue" is added at the end of the book.

函三为一歌并图

The Song and Diagram of Three-Yuan-in-One

天地人三元，每元六十年，三六一百八十年，此寿得于天。天本全付与，于人或自偏。全之有其法，奈何世罕传。函三为一图，妙探太极先。外圆而内方，一坤与一乾。定体凝坤象，妙用周乾圆。寿年在其间，得之本自然。一岁加一点，渐比乔彭肩。未悟参赞法，所点恐莫全。此书神仙诀，识者作寿仙。颜朱发长绿，髓满骨且坚。岂特点尽图，天地相周旋。

The three Yuan of the heaven, the earth and the human-being, each endowed with 60 years and amounted to 180 years, is the lifespan blessed by natural law to all the people in the world. But some can not enjoy it because of certain wrong doings and the methods to correct can be rarely found and handed down. The diagram of Three-Yuan-in-One is a good exploration of the profoundness of Taiji. It is round outside and square inside, representing Qian and Kun[①]. The manifestations of Kun are presented in the middle

---

① Qian and Kun: Qian, one of the Eight Diagrams, denoting the heaven; Kun, one of the Eight Diagrams, denoting the earth.

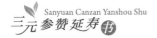

and the movement of Qian is circulating magically around. The longevity is determined by these diagrams and bestowed to people by the natural law. With time passing year by year, people grow older gradually and they can enjoy a long lifespan just as Qiao Song and Peng Zu[①]. But it may be hard to attain one's longevity without reading and understanding this book thoroughly. This book is something like a pithy formula which can help people enjoy a long lifespan like immortals by keeping people young and strong. So just follow the natural law as showed by the diagram and live to one's full age as a result of the interaction between the heaven and the earth.

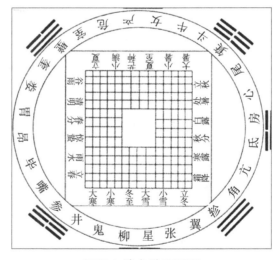

行天之健应地无疆图

(The Diagram of Following the Law of Heaven and Conforming to the Infinite Earth)

---

① Qiao Song refers to two immortals in the ancient time, who are named Wang Ziqiao and Chi Songzi respectively. Peng Zu refers to a legendary figure of Taoism in the ancient time who lived 800 years.

还元图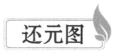

The Diagram of Restoring Vitality

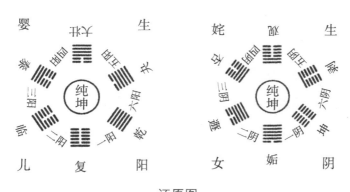

还原图

（ The Diagram of Restoring Vitality ）

乾，阳刚也，生意本具，一旦为阴柔乘之，为姤、为遁、为否、为观、为剥，剥极而为坤。坤，纯阴也，阴极则主杀矣。苟知所复则硕果不食。阴极而阳，静极而动，生意又勃然矣。

Qian（an ancient Chinese philosophic term, often used together with Kun to refer one of the two opposite sides like yang, or heaven）corresponds to masculine in property and is characteristic of all living things. Just as what is illustrated in the first graphical representation, once Qian is subjugated by

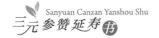
femininity, it starts to transform and turns into the hexagram of Gou, then the hexagram of Dun, then the hexagram of Pi, then the hexagram of Guan, then the hexagram of Bo, and finally the hexagram of Kun. Kun（an ancient Chinese philosophic term, often used together with Qian to refer one of the two opposite sides like yin, or earth）corresponds to extreme feminine in property and governs the ending of all living things. The eventual result needs to be preserved if one knows all things go in a circular order just as the big fruit being kept uneaten. Extreme yin can transform into yang, extreme stillness can transform into movement, so everything can start a new circle and restore vigorous life again.

坤，阴也，阴极阳复。阴，人欲也。阳，天理也。以理制欲，于是阳长阴消，患迷复耳。苟不迷焉，复而临，临而泰，泰而大壮，大壮而夬。夬，决也，决则纯乾，可复行天之健，与天同寿矣。

Kun pertains to yin in property and extreme yin brings on the re-occurrence of yang. Yin corresponds to human desire and yang to heavenly principle. When the human desire is restrained by heavenly principle, yang begins to wax and yin begins to wane, which may lead to confusion instead of clear perception. If this transformation is not confused, it turns into the hexagram of Fu, then the hexagram of Lin, then the hexagram of Tai, then the hexagram of Dazhuang, and then the hexagram of Guai. Guai is synonymous with the Chinese character "Jue", which is followed by the hexagram of Qian. This indicates that the health of heaven can be restored and the longevity can be achieved.

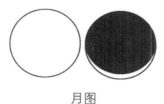

月图

（Diagram of Moon Waxing and Waning）

道心泯而人心胜，则自望至晦之月也。

The fact that moral principle is surpassed by human desire is just like the moon turning from the full to the waning state on the last day of a lunar month.

人欲尽而天理还，则自旦至望之月也。

The fact that heavenly principle restores and human desire reduces is just like the moon turning from the waning state on the first day of a lunar month to the full state.